10 0555695 3

KU-272-137

WITHDRAWN

The Globalisation of Nur

The Globalisation of Nursing

Edited by

VERENA TSCHUDIN

Editor, *Nursing Ethics*
Director, International Centre for Nursing Ethics,
University of Surrey

and

ANNE J DAVIS

Professor Emerita, University of California, San Francisco
Emerita, Nagano College of Nursing, Japan

UNIVERSITY OF NOTTINGHAM
SCHOOL OF NURSING &
MIDWIFERY
DERBYSHIRE ROYAL INFIRMARY
LONDON ROAD DERBY
DE1 2QY

Foreword by

CHRISTINE HANCOCK

Director, Oxford Health Alliance
former President, International Council of Nurses

Radcliffe Publishing
Oxford • New York

Radcliffe Publishing Ltd
18 Marcham Road
Abingdon
Oxon OX14 1AA
United Kingdom

www.radcliffe-oxford.com

Electronic catalogue and worldwide online ordering facility.

© 2008 Verena Tschudin and Anne J Davis

Verena Tschudin and Anne J Davis have asserted their right under the Copyright,
Designs and Patents Act 1998 to be identified as the authors of this work.

All rights reserved. No part of this publication may be reproduced, stored in a
retrieval system or transmitted, in any form or by any means, electronic, mechanical,
photocopying, recording or otherwise, without the prior permission of the copyright
owner.

British Library Cataloguing in Publication Data

A catalogue record for this book is available from the British Library.

ISBN-13: 978 184619 149 7

Typeset by Pindar NZ, Auckland, New Zealand
Printed and bound by TJI Digital, Padstow, Cornwall, UK

Contents

Foreword

This book on globalisation is a welcome addition to the nursing literature for professional nurses working internationally and at home. Additionally, it has some important messages for others in the healthcare services and for the public at large. The topics included cover a wide range of issues that impact on nurses, the nursing profession, and all those who receive nursing care.

Such a book brings to both practicing nurses and students a wider view of our nursing world and demonstrates how interconnected we really are in so many ways. Some of the topics will be familiar while others may not be so, but all are important for us to understand in the provision of care to people from diverse cultures and as we live and work with international colleagues. The reality of nurse migration has many complex dimensions for all involved. This issue, like several others addressed here, is not only of professional concern but touches on human rights in a general way. Sometimes our first response to any issue does not take all the factors into account. This book considers many of them, questions practices and policies at many levels, and shows some innovative means of care and education. That is why I urge you to read and reflect on all the global themes in this book. You will enjoy it and be the wiser for your effort.

Christine Hancock
Director, Oxford Health Alliance
former President, International Council of Nurses
July 2008

List of contributors

Helen Allan

I have always been interested in the social side of nursing delivery and healthcare policy. I became interested in globlisation a few years ago when I was asked to complete a qualitative study into the experiences of overseas nurses. I realised that, as a professional group, nurses in the United Kingdom (UK) were largely unaware of the effects of workforce changes on individual overseas nurses and that our ethnocentric attitudes might render negative their experiences of living and working in the UK. I continue to write and research in the area of social and emotional aspects of nursing and workforce issues while working at the Centre for Research in Nursing and Midwifery Education at the University of Surrey.

Wendy Austin

My work in health ethics began, in a concentrated way, in the late 1990s when I received an incredible gift: a research fellowship to study international bioethics. During the time of the fellowship, I was concurrently working to achieve designation for my Faculty of Nursing at the University of Alberta, Canada, as a World Health Collaborating Centre in mental health. This exciting time shaped my need to understand how to be an ethical nurse in our global community. A Canada Research Chair in Relational Ethics has allowed me to pursue this and other questions related to ethical practice.

Sylvia Bertram

In 1986, I was asked to teach a nursing class that included ethics at Samuel Merritt College. I knew very little about ethics at the time, so I started a life-long quest for more information and a deeper understanding of ethics. Fortunately, part of my education included working with Dr Edmund Pellegrino. For the past few years, I have used ethics as a base for discussing subjects that often polarise people because of the strong beliefs they hold. Since international recruiting of nurses prompts much heated discussion, I wanted to use ethical principles as a foundation for that discussion.

Mark Chamberlain

Since qualifying as a registered mental health nurse, I have been working with people suffering from dementia and those who, because of mental illness, have been diverted away from the criminal justice system. Recognising the increasing importance that human rights have for those working in healthcare, I left nursing briefly to study for an LLM in International Human Rights Law at the University of Essex. In addition, my interest in human rights has led me to supervise and monitor elections in the UK, Central America, the Balkans and Ukraine.

Freida S Chavez

I am a lecturer in global health and international nursing at the Lawrence S Bloomberg Faculty of Nursing, University of Toronto, Canada. It has been great to start the journey of building global citizenship through education by formally integrating global health in our nursing curriculum. Designing and teaching two global health courses in the second entry BScN programme, which are described in Chapter 16, is very exciting. I do this work in partnership with colleagues globally, including Aboriginal and First Nations in Canada, Africa and India.

Anne J Davis

After receiving the Kennedy Fellowship at Harvard in 1976, my teaching and research focused on ethics at the University of California, San Francisco (UCSF), where I worked for 34 years. I was invited to many countries to lecture and con-duct research. On retirement from UCSF, I taught at Nagano College of Nursing, Japan, for six years. During that time I published several books, over 200 articles, and numerous book chapters. I received many awards, including an honorary DSc degree from Emory University, Atlanta, and the first ANA Human Rights Award. Now my work continues to focus on nursing ethics and human rights.

Leyla Dinç

During the first five years of my career, while working as a clinical nurse, I realised that professional nursing practice demands not only knowledge and technical skills but also ethical principles. I am now a faculty member in the School of Nursing at Hacettepe University, Ankara, and, through teaching ethics as part of a nursing course in my institution, I have become increasingly interested in nursing ethics. My major interests are ethics education, and the impact of culture and politics on healthcare. I serve as an editorial board member of *Nursing Ethics* and on the Ethics Commission of Hacettepe University Senate.

Anastasia A Fisher

My early career experiences as a psychiatric nurse working with persons who live with serious mental illnesses, together with my doctoral education at UCSF, where I was privileged to meet and study ethics with Dr Anne Davis, were influential in shaping my interest in the ethical foundations of nursing practice and human rights. My current community-based participatory research programme with Dr Diane Hatton focuses on healthcare access and healthcare justice for incarcerated women.

Denise Gastaldo

My scholarship explores the politics of health practices and knowledge production from a global health perspective. My research focuses on gender and migration as social determinants of health, as well as power relations in health promotion and healthcare. In recent years, I have undertaken research in Canada, Brazil and Spain, and co-edited two books on qualitative methodologies in Ibero-America. I am currently the coordinator of the International Nursing PhD Collaboration, which includes programmes from Australia, Canada, Mexico and Spain.

Mary Tod Gray

I have been drawn to nursing ethics through two particular interests: my research in the philosophy of addictions and my perception of the undermining of ethical standards by national political leaders. The first interest led me to question the moral dimensions of addiction from multiple perspectives: those of the individual, of nurses, and of a global healthcare environment in which addictions both affect and reflect ethical behaviours and commitments at many levels. The second interest led me to question how political leaders perceive the moral commitments of their roles and, in particular, how nursing leaders in education experience those ethical dimensions in their role.

Diane C Hatton

Over the years, my research and clinical interests have been in the area of community/public health nursing, with a special focus on vulnerable populations. During my doctoral studies at UCSF, I had the good fortune of studying with Dr Anne Davis and developing an appreciation of the relevance of ethics to my work. My current community-based participatory research with Dr Anastasia Fisher focuses on healthcare access and healthcare justice for incarcerated women.

Tova Hendel

I have for many years worked in senior managerial positions in education, in acute care hospitals and the community. Concurrently, for the last 20 years, I have been a faculty member at the Department of Nursing, Tel Aviv University, Israel. My publications focus on subjects related to nursing management (leadership styles, conflict management, interdisciplinary collaboration, organisational values) and nursing education (preparation for managerial roles, students' value sets). As Head of the Baccalaureate programme for the last six years, I have signed a growing number of translated transcripts for nursing graduates who wish to emigrate, a task that is frustrating and upsetting.

Susan J Henly

I am a quantitative methodologist, educator and nurse with American Indian health research, teaching and practice experience. It is a great privilege for me to serve in the research training programmes of American Indian nurses. May our experiences create a positive chapter in the story of American Indian education.

Leroi Henry

I am a research fellow at the Faculty of Health and Social Care of the Open University, currently working on a project documenting the contribution to the NHS of South Asian-trained geriatricians and exploring their experiences over the previous 50 years. Earlier I worked on the Researching Equal Opportunities for Internationally Recruited Nurses and Other Healthcare Professionals (REOH) project, which explored the experiences of migrant nurses in the UK. Other research interests focus on the interplay between identity, migration and international development, and have included exploring the roles of diasporas in development, and the relationship between ethnicity and indigenous development in Africa.

Miriam J Hirschfeld

My interest in ethics began in my teens when first reading about the medical experiments in the German concentration camps and the experiments during the Japanese invasion of China, as well as when, later, as a young nurse, I saw the effects of the atomic bomb in Hiroshima. When I started nursing school, I wondered where the nurses had been in those horrific situations and if they had had the courage to object. One of my early research studies focused on force-feeding patients with dementia, as part of a large international study. In the years since, I have worked for the World Health Organization and have had ample opportunity to question what 'ethical behaviour' is, and how universal or culture specific it might be.

Dominique Le Touze

Working as a researcher on a mental health project for the East Timor Commission for Reception, Truth and Reconciliation, I became interested in the important link between health and human rights. I was able to pursue this as a volunteer for Amnesty International when I worked on a report for nurses and midwives, examining ethics and human rights issues. Ensuring that healthcare systems continue to uphold ethical principles and practices, and that healthcare workers are supported to do this, remains a key part of my current work in public health for the UK NHS.

Gustav Moyo

Following graduation from nursing school in Tanzania, I was posted to work in a remote district hospital, where I gained immensely useful experience in how to deal with the high expectations of clients using health services in an environment with limited resources. This stimulated my initial serious interest in ethics, as I was often faced with dilemmas of providing services that are not traditionally regarded as a nurse's responsibility. I was involved in HIV and AIDS studies conducted in Tanzania in collaboration with institutions from developed countries, and this involvement further stimulated several moral questions, particularly in relation to consent and access to treatment, and care and support for poor study participants. My current work in the Tanzania Nursing Council provides a different version of moral and ethical challenges: overworked nurses often succumb to mistakes and the public expects us to discipline these nurses.

Lee Anne Nichols

My family is Ghormley and Foreman of Tahlequah, Oklahoma, and I am a citizen of the Cherokee Nation. My programme of research involves American Indian families with children with disabilities. I teach community health nursing at the University of Tulsa. My life goal is to serve and improve the health of American Indians. It is an honour to be a part of this book.

Elizabeth Niven

My interest in ethics was sparked by the visit to New Zealand of Alastair Campbell in the early 1980s. I well remember a colleague's irritation at Professor Campbell's failure to provide clear answers to all the tricky questions, and my struggle to communicate how limiting such an approach would be. I have been in nursing education for 20 years and have maintained my interest in ethics during that time, learning, teaching, writing and consulting. I find ethics one of those fields where learning more only uncovers what there still is to learn.

Judy Goforth Parker

I have taught as a professor at East Central University, Ada, Oklahoma, for the past 24 years. During that time, I have taught courses in community health and the childbearing family, served as a member of several committees, and developed the first blended course in our undergraduate nursing programme. I am a member of the American Public Health Association. I have served as an elected official in my tribe, the Chickasaw Nation, for the past 13 years. I am active in national work for tribes as I help to combat the diabetic epidemic. I have served as a member of the Tribal Leaders Diabetes Committee for nine years. My major interests are related to nursing, diabetes, and the Chickasaw Nation.

Elizabeth Peter

I am Associate Professor and Associate Dean, Academic Programs, Lawrence S Bloomberg Faculty of Nursing, and member, Joint Centre for Bioethics, University of Toronto, Canada. I consider myself to be a highly fortunate individual in that I have been able to pursue two of my academic passions – nursing and philosophy – simultaneously. My students challenge me to keep nursing ethics relevant to practice and policy, both locally and globally. I write widely in the field of nursing ethics and address ethical issues in home and community care.

Richard Rowson

I wrote course units on moral philosophy at the Open University before moving to the University of Glamorgan, in Wales. As well as lecturing in moral and political philosophy, I work with practitioners in medicine, nursing, social work, education and the police. My assignments have included: tutor in ethics, St Mary's Medical School, London; member of the ethics committee, Royal College of Nursing; consultant on police ethics, UK Home Office; writing teaching programmes for nurses and the police; advising universities on their ethics policies; and contributing to radio and television programmes. My latest book is *Working Ethics*, published in 2006.

Faye Thompson

I studied philosophy and the humanities as an undergraduate in Australia, and after gaining more than 20 years' experience as a midwife and educator, I now lecture on and conduct research into the ethics of clinical practice. As a feminist, I seek to unite morality and personal interest so that individuals, and in particular childbearing women, are not subordinated in healthcare practices. Hearing mothers' and midwives' narratives enabled me to identify for the first time a midwifery ethic that had emerged from within the practice. Together with recent media reports on whistleblowing in healthcare settings, this has led me to question the impact of disclosure of mistakes and unethical behaviour on individuals, and explore how our systems can promote the benefits of reporting and discussion.

Verena Tschudin

After many years of active nursing, most of it in oncology, the area of ethics presented itself as a natural follow-on. The journal *Nursing Ethics*, which I have edited since its start, offered a sharp learning curve in many ways, and also the opportunity to write, speak and travel widely. The International Centre for Nursing Ethics (ICNE) at the University of Surrey, UK, has become a hub for various international activities and interests, and enables me, as its director, to develop the wider views of nursing that I believe will need to be tackled in the future of the profession.

Huey-Ming Tzeng

I became interested in ethics when Taiwan was attacked by severe acute respiratory syndrome (SARS) in 2003. Since then I have been concerned about the safety of patients and clinical staff when delivering healthcare across the care continuum. Related ethical issues are indeed linked to global health and the globalisation movement. In the past 10 years, I took both macro- and micro-approaches to address healthcare quality issues. My research areas involve patient safety in hospitals; healthcare management and delivery systems; religions, cultures and care quality; newly emerging infectious diseases and global health, and research methodology. Promoting safe hospital stays is my current research theme at the University of Michigan School of Nursing.

Nurith Wagner

My interest in ethics goes back to my nursing school days when paternalism was practised toward not only patients but nurses, too. Since 2002, I have chaired the Israeli Nurses Association's Ethics Bureau. I developed an ethical decision-making simulation game that is used for nursing education across the country and also for the development of ethics forums in different health services across Israel. I am a member of the Israeli government Bioethics Committee and serve on the Hadassah Medical Organization Institutional Research Board. I am also a member of the Ministry of Health accessibility committee for promotion of access to healthcare for disabled people, and a member of Machsom (checkpoints) Watch, the Israeli women's organisation against the occupation and for human-rights. In 2007, I received the ICNE Human Rights and Nursing Award.

James Welsh

My work at Amnesty International, a departure from my training as a virologist, encompasses all aspects of the intersection between health and human rights. The right to health is increasingly seen as an important international human-rights issue, and is a major concern in my own work. I have a particular interest in health professionals as defenders of human rights, and in the role of ethics as a protective tool for both health personnel and the public.

Chang-Yi Yin

I have been interested in and researched the subjects of Chinese history, area and culture studies, theology, medicine and psychology. As a social activist, I have led and been the leader of several social actions in Taiwan. At the beginning of the SARS outbreak in Taiwan in 2003, my inner voice urged me to study human responses to help people survive SARS and any future newly-emerging infectious diseases. Promoting global health is the theme of my recent research at the Department of History, Chinese Culture University, Taipei, Taiwan.

SECTION 1

Setting the global scene

1

Introduction and the topic of globalisation

Anne J Davis and Verena Tschudin

INTRODUCTION

This book is a compilation and expansion of papers presented at the annual conference of the International Centre for Nursing Ethics (ICNE) held in the summer of 2006 at the University of Surrey, Guildford, UK. The topic – globalisation – while not new, is especially important in these early years of the twenty-first century, and this examination of selected aspects of globalisation that impact nursing and healthcare is timely for nurses in every country, whether economically developed or developing.

The themes of these papers range from a discussion of globalisation as a concept and a reality, and its impact on areas of the globe, the health of human populations and the practice of nursing, to other broadly conceptualised papers on such questions as the right to healthcare and a global basis for nursing ethics, to more specific problems such as addiction, nurse migration, women prisoners, nursing standards and terrorism, all of which have a global dimension. Some of the chapters provide information from one country that can be extended to the global community. These latter chapters focus on such diverse topics as nursing education, patient safety and ethnicity in a globally connected world. What results is a rich mixture of ideas to ponder and discuss, for surely some, if not all, of these issues will impact healthcare and every nurse everywhere on our planet.

While we do not think of ourselves as technological determinists, we are aware of technology that can be used by health professionals across national borders to assist with health-related issues, specific diagnoses, and with global plans for dealing with these issues. In addition, the worldwide web is full of information regarding clinical positions in many countries. For example, Qatar, a small country in the Middle East rich in gas and oil deposits, has pages of such information. One particular nursing problem in many countries is the ability to prepare teachers of nurses. We know that for years nursing texts written in English have been translated into other languages for use elsewhere. Web-based and distance-learning devices in nursing are now used frequently and are often preferable. Nurse teachers can now be in one part of the world and teach in another in an interactive fashion. This is called teaching in 'real time'.

Along with such advancements, we have also witnessed the tragic global spread of HIV/AIDS. We read about possible pandemics of bird flu and other contagious diseases. Later chapters in this book address some aspects of these health problems, made more complex by our globalised world situation. The spread of contagious diseases is certainly an example of how globalisation is affecting diseases and nursing.

Therefore, how nurses are taught, how they work, where they work and with whom they work are no longer just local realities. Globalisation has changed that forever. The type of patient nurses care for has also changed and will change even more in the future. The chapters later in this book on how nurses are to be prepared and to cope in a globalised world discuss these realities. No nurse and no healthcare system will go untouched by these profound changes.

GLOBALISATION: THEN AND NOW

Much has been written about globalisation, covering a wide range of topics from its benefits to the negative aspects of this development. While the reality of globalisation is not entirely new, the word as it is used today has become commonplace only in the last few decades. It entered the dictionary in 1961, has been used by economists since 1981, and entered the public's consciousness in the late 1990s. Best-sellers on the topic, such as Thomas L. Friedman's *The World is Flat* (2005), now translated into numerous languages, helped the public gain a better understanding of globalisation. The academic literature is vast and the topic so important that universities – such as Yale in the United States (US), Warwick in the UK, and the Copenhagen Business School in Denmark – have established centres for the study of globalisation.

Some authors think that the rapid integration of the world's economy that occurred in the nineteenth and twentieth centuries is a new global reality and surely a defining issue as we move further into the twenty-first century (Bhagwati 2004). The words 'global' and 'globalisation' are sometimes confused and, while they do share the same root, they also have somewhat different meanings. 'Global' means involving the entire world, while 'globalisation' has come to refer to a process of increasing global connections, interdependence and integration, especially in the economic arena, but also affecting cultural, social, political, ecological and technological aspects of life.

For some time the concept of globalisation has been controversial. The reasons for this indicate the complexity and uncertainty of the effect that globalisation is having and will continue to have on people around the globe. Without knowing full details of the future, we do know that globalisation will continue to impact much of our daily lives in where we live and who our close neighbours are; who works for whom; what we buy to eat and wear, and who gets what kind and amount of healthcare.

While the future may be somewhat unclear, the past gives us details showing that some powerful individuals and groups have exploited vulnerable people. Not all such exploitation occurred in the West, although much – including slavery, indentured servitude and trafficking of people, especially of women and children – did happen there. For some people, the most important value is the accumulation of money. These are only the most blatant reasons why some people view globalisation not only as an economic trend but also as a moral issue involving human rights.

This controversy is due in large part to the gap between what globalisation could do to help people to raise their living standards, especially poor people in poor countries, and the realities of how globalisation has been managed, which at times has been devastating in poor countries. The familiar problem of the 'ethical ought' and the 'is of reality' that we know so well when we focus on ethical issues in healthcare is well demonstrated in this economic development.

Joseph Stiglitz (2003), a Nobel Prize winner in economics with firsthand experience at the World Bank and the International Monetary Fund, as well as having been economic adviser to the Clinton administration, says that globalisation can be a force for good, with the potential to enrich everyone in the world, especially the poor, but this will take fundamental reforms in the international economic architecture, the system by which the international economic and financial systems are governed. To benefit people in developing countries, globalisation will need to become more humane, effective, and equitable. Paul Farmer *et al.* (2003) working with TB patients in Haiti, Peru and Russia is a remarkable model for humane globalisation. He maintains that making social and economic rights a reality is the key goal for health and human rights in the twenty-first century.

Globalisation is not a new idea or reality, but the way the word 'globalisation' is now used is fairly new, and reforms are surely needed to make it a fair and just system. In fact, some models of globalisation reach back into history to include war and conquest, ancient trade routes, explorations over lands and sea, as well as diplomatic relations. We may have forgotten that the Vikings entered Dublin in the ninth century, while in the east, Genghis Khan (1162–1227) established the most extensive empire ever recorded in history that included parts of Asia,

Europe and Africa. The Mongols ruled, or at least briefly conquered, large parts of modern-day China, Mongolia, Russia, Azerbaijan, Armenia, Georgia, Iraq, Iran, Turkey, Kazakhstan, Kyrgyzstan, Uzbekistan, Pakistan, Tajikistan, Afghanistan, Turkmenistan, Moldova, South Korea, North Korea, and Kuwait (Weatherford 2004). The famous Spice Route and Silk Road, somewhat less aggressive approaches to globalisation, made important socio-economic and cultural connections across space and peoples. While globalisation as a concept and reality is not new, it is vital to realise today that its ramifications are potentially one hundred per cent global and immediate, owing to technological developments in transportation and communication. Time and space have been forever altered, and the globe has become smaller but not less complex.

WHAT IS NEEDED IN A GLOBALISED WORLD

Because globalisation, whatever form it takes, impacts so many people in so many places, and this impact will influence, if not determine, the health and well-being of most, and perhaps all, human populations on the globe, it is worthy of our serious attention. Both as citizens and as nurses, we need to explore the health and human-rights dimension that globalisation brings about in our world, sometimes referred to as a village, so as to understand our professional responsibilities. These responsibilities go beyond understanding the basic issues to include possible actions we can take to influence policy and events before they occur, and work to improve the outcome of new policies as well as the ones already in place. Gandhi said, 'Almost everything you do will be insignificant, but it is important that you do it.' We as editors believe and value this idea very strongly. It is very easy to become overwhelmed by all the many serious problems in the world to the extent that individual nurses do nothing. Yet individuals and groups can make a difference in many ways. All of us need to think and act globally, with realistic expectations, and we need to work in groups of nurses and others concerned about the state of our planet.

The complexities and uncertainties of globalisation are grounded in notions of human rights and justice that are discussed in some of the chapters. The global public good depends on these basic and most fundamental ethical principles.

While it is extremely difficult for most individuals to have any impact on the development of globalisation, it is possible for informed individuals working in groups and through various organisations to make a difference on specific aspects of this movement. Jagdish Bhagwati (2004) believes that globalisation has a human face, i.e. that this is not some amorphous force out there, but individuals and groups of individuals that affect economic changes. Globalisation has great potential to create a better life for all people everywhere, especially the poor, but it has not fully realised this potential to date. However, not eveyone agrees with Bhagwati, in that they view globalisation as developed by the interaction of governmental policies and multinational corporations well beyond the reach of most people to influence in any major way.

Not only is a change in mind-set needed in the goverance of economic institutions, national governments and international policy-making organisations, but individuals and the groups with which they work to affect change need fresh ways of thinking about the globe and globalisation and their role in it.

Miriam Hirschfeld, who disagrees with Bhagwati, reminds us in the next chapter that it is unlikely an individual can effect change, but we (the editors) think it is possible for individuals working through organisations to make a difference. These might include watchdog groups, such as Amnesty International or Human Rights Watch, and professional groups, such as national nursing associations or other professional groups for nurses (*see also* Chapter 20). The US online group, MoveOn (www.moveon.org), a political information and action group, reaches great numbers of people, and helps them to act in an informed and timely fashion on specific issues, often before national or state government decision-making bodies do.

The one thing most needed is being informed about the new world order. This includes more fully inderstanding several facts.

- ❑ Globalisation is here to stay.
- ❑ Globalisation affects health status and healthcare for individuals, population groups, nations, regions and the globe.
- ❑ Globalisation impacts nursing at all levels and in all places.
- ❑ There are many benefits to be gained from globalisation.
- ❑ There are also numerous problems with globalisation, not always acknowledged by people in countries that currently benefit from this economic arrangement.
- ❑ Globalisation needs to be undertstood in relation to historical social class and gender issues.
- ❑ Globalisation depends on multinational companies which, according to some, have replaced national governments and control the ecnonomy of nations in a transnational mode.

SOCIO-ECONOMIC STATUS AND GENDER ISSUES: POVERTY AND WOMEN

Numerous authors, including those cited in this chapter, fear that globalisation will widen the gap between the haves and the have-nots. Some see this economic-based development as a major means of continuing prosperity and the status quo in the developed world, and thereby maintaining massive poverty in the developing world. This picture is painted by some analysists in various hues of darkness, but all are gloomy and akin to Francisco Goya's (1746–1828) paintings in the series on the Disasters of War. Some people think that war has been extended to include aggressive actions against: terrorists, drugs, and poor people, therefore this is an appropriate reference point here (Farmer 2003; Sachs 2005).

Other analyses view globalisation in a different light, with brighter colours, and see the cooperation and interlaced nature of the global economy as a major means to lift poor countries out of their poverty by improving standards of living, life expectancy, healthcare delivery, literacy rates, and so on. Some say a change is needed that includes a reshaping of the present set of doctrines imposed by the International Monetary Fund and the World Bank. Some refer to this as market fundamentalism, while others call it the Washington Consensus policies, which assume that one set of policies fits all, having been imposed by international financial institutions (Stiglitz 2003).

Globalisation is a complex topic with multiple dimensions but this discussion is limited to two such topics: poverty and gender. Being poor makes it difficult to be healthy; poverty involves being unable to meet basic needs, including obtaining preventive and curative healthcare. Women have a major influence on their families, and their decisions impact their own health status as well as that of their children and their husbands.

GLOBALISATION AND POVERTY

We all know that social class has an impact on the health status of individuals, while a country's economy – including the allocation of resources that are always scarce even in rich countries – determines the type and amount of healthcare available to its citizens. The number of people around the globe living on less than USD1 a day is an appalling statistic in the twenty-first century, especially when affluence and waste best describe what happens in other areas of the globe. Multiple factors come together to create ongoing poverty: the lack of infrastructure and an undeveloped industrial base; the lack of education necessary to obtain the most rudimentary skills of reading and writing; low per-capita income; lack of foreign investments, and the legacy of imperialism. These continued through much of the twentieth century, taking from economically poor countries to benefit wealthy countries. It is relevant here to mention that many countries, especially in Africa and to some extent in Asia, are only recently independent, e.g. India 1947, Egypt 1951, Ghana 1957, Nigeria 1960, Kenya 1963, Botswana 1966, Zimbabwe 1980, Namibia 1990. All of this social and economic change occurred within our (the editors') lifetime. Most of these nations were part of the British empire and even today have kept English law, which may not always fit their cultures.

Other factors that maintained the economic status quo in poor countries include: inadequate leadership at the national level leading to the inability to develop a world view that goes beyond one's family, clan, tribe, or religious group; and the ability or incentive to think of the common good for the nation, the region, the world. In his autobiography, Nelson Mandela discussed the moment when he first thought of the world beyond his own tribe (1995).

Many of us are not heroes like Nelson Mandela, but rather still think in terms of our own more narrow sphere of life, work and influence. Technological developments and issues such as global warming and poverty are forcing us to think physically and psychologically in these larger categories beyond our immediate lives. Not thinking about, discussing or acting to influence are reactions that can be found in many, if not most, countries, whether developed or developing, as well as those more or less static, or in economic decline. Such shortcomings are regularly discussed in quality and popular newspapers and magazines as well as in the professional literature, including that published by the United Nations (UN).

How we conceptualise poverty is a central factor in any discussion of globalisation. The famous economist, Amartya Sen (1999) says that there are good reasons for thinking of poverty as a deprivation of basic capabilities and not just low income. Deprivation of elementary capabilities can be reflected in premature mortality, significant undernourishment (especially of children), persistent morbidity, widespread illiteracy and other failures. Such a view of poverty is based on an innate freedom, which is the ability to survive rather than succumb to premature mortality. This perspective is similar to the often-voiced nursing concern for quality of life, and widens the discussion from a focus on poverty and wealth, where the emphasis is on income only. This broader approach finds its roots in Aristotle's focus on flourishing and capacity (McKeon 2001), and with Adam Smith's analysis of necessities and conditions of living (Smith & Krueger 2003).

GLOBALISATION AND GENDER

Gender has come to represent an important element in understanding poverty and the impact of globalisation. Some groups of women have received more attention in the literature because they are the ones travelling the globe in search of work. Annually, millions of women leave developing countries for jobs in homes, nurseries and brothels in developed countries. According to Barbara Ehrenreich and Arlie Russell Hochschild, this enormous transfer of labour eases a 'care deficit' in rich countries while creating one back home. Information on legal migrants is available, but not on illegal migrants. However, experts report that the latter group travel in equal if not greater numbers. These same experts speak of the 'feminisation of migration' (Ehrenreich & Hochschild 2002, pp. 285–6). In examining the dynamics of globalisation, other authors explore gender, race, class inequality, migration, citizenship and the politics of social control in care work, which they think plays a pivotal role in accentuating gender and global inequalities. The population trend at present is to move from south to north, east to west and from country to city.

Globalisation concerns itself with the upper, not the lower, circuits of global capital, hence the underside of outsourcing and cheap service work is obscured. Mary Zimmerman *et al.* (2006) discuss the commodification of care, and include a chapter focusing on this process in nursing. Our world, including nursing, is increasingly shaped by mass migration and economic exchange.

In exploring other dimensions of gender and globalisation, Deborah Brandt (2002) asked the simple question 'Where does our food come from?', and traced women's work in the tomato market as it travelled north from Mexico, where women picked and packed the produce for shipment to the US. There, women worked in fast-food chains selling hamburgers with tomatoes. In Canadian supermarkets, women sold tomatoes from Mexico. The northward journey from field to table reveals the true heart of corporate globalisation, and low-paid women are at the centre of this heart.

In the book, *Gender, Globalization, and Democratization* (Kelly *et al.* 2001) the authors dramatically make the point that the migration of women in large numbers is global. They describe women in Oceania, Europe, Africa, Mexico, India and East Asia in relation to globalisation and democratisation to illustrate the many issues and problems involved. However, the authors also remind us that women are not only passive victims in 'global factories'. Recent studies show that women in South Korea, the Philippines and South Africa fight against the practices of wage dumping, deskilling and other tactics of transnational corporations (Ward and Pyle 1995).

Issues of social class, poverty and gender inequalities are among those addressed either directly or indirectly in the chapters that follow. Other global issues discussed in this book raise questions of human rights with embedded notions of obligations, especially those of wealthy nation to poor countries. All these global issues, which impact health, healthcare, nursing, and in the final analysis each one of us, raise a plethra of ethical and policy questions.

CONCLUSION AND A BEGINNING

We, the editors, view this book as a beginning of the further education of student nurses, practising nurses and other health professionals on the subject of globalisation and its numerous impacts, not only on nursing and health but on the multifaceted lives of individuals around the globe. There are gaps in this effort that need exploration and development in the near future if the informed dialogue is to continue. For example, this book has only one chapter from a developing country while other chapters, in discussing migration of nurses, do touch on developing countries' issues of health status and health personnel. We offer this beginning in the spirit of international colleagueship, and we urge you to think about these issues as a citizen of the world who has special and urgently needed knowledge and skills. Welcome to our shared globalised and troubled world, a world in which Peter Singer teaches us that we need to take an ethical perspective on globalisation (2002). We entirely agree with his position.

REFERENCES

Bhagwati J. In Defence of Globalization. New York: Oxford University Press; 2004.

Brandt D. Tangled Routes: women, work and globalization on the tomato trail. New York: Rowman & Littlefield; 2002.

Ehrenreich B, Hochschild AR. Global Women: nannies, maids and sex workers in the new economy. New York: Henry Holt; 2002.

Farmer P. Pathologies of Power: health, human rights and the new war on the poor. Berkeley, CA: University of California Press; 2003.

Friedman TL. The World is Flat: a brief history of the twenty-first century. New York: Farrar, Straus & Giroux; 2005.

Kelly RM, Bayes JH, Hawkesworth ME, Young B, editors. Gender, Globalization and Democratization. New York: Rowman & Littlefield; 2001.

Mandela N. Long Walk to Freedom: the autobiography of Nelson Mandela. Boston, MA: Back Bay Books; 1995.

McKeon R, editor. The Basic Works of Aristotle. New York: Modern Library; 2001.

Sachs JD. The End of Poverty: economic possibilities in our time. New York: Penguin Press; 2005.

Sen A. Development as Freedom. New York: Random House; 1999.

Singer P. One World: the ethics of globalization. New Haven, CT: Yale Univeristy Press; 2002.

Smith A. The Wealth of Nations. New York: Bantam Books, 2003.

Stiglitz JE. Globalization and its Discontent. New York: Norton; 2003.

Ward K, Pyle JL. Gender, Industrialization, Transnational Corporations and Development: an overview of trends and patterns. In: Bose CE, Acosta-Belen E, editors. Women in the Latin American Development Process. Phildelphia: Temple University Press; 1995. pp. 37–64.

Weatherford J. Genghis Khan and the Making of the Modern World. New York: Three Rivers Press; 2004.

Zimmerman MK, Litt JS, Bose CE. Global Dimensions of Gender and Carework. Stanford, CA: Stanford University Press; 2006.

2

Globalisation: good or bad, for whom?

Miriam J Hirschfeld

DEFINING GLOBALISATION: THE POLITICAL AND ECONOMIC CONTEXT

'Globalisation is the process by which the experience of everyday life, marked by the diffusion of commodities and ideas, is becoming standardised around the world' (*Encyclopedia Britannica* 2002). The defining feature of globalisation is the worldwide integration of economic and financial sectors, which was made possible by three crucial developments: technological progress, geopolitical changes and the dominant ideology of regulation by the market. A complimentary definition by Rhys Jenkins (2004, p. 1) defines globalisation as 'a process of greater integration within the world economy through movements of goods and services, capital, technology and (to a lesser extent) labour, which lead increasingly to economic decisions being influenced by global conditions.'

Without the technology of the Internet and means of rapid communication, such as email, globalisation is not imaginable. Without the geopolitical changes following the demise of the Soviet Union and the opening of borders, which led to the widely accepted belief that markets regulate themselves and free market economy is the best system, globalisation as we know it would not have been possible.

On the one hand, globalisation unifies the world, but, on the other hand, as the importance of human and social capital is often ignored and concern for the well-being of people is ranking low in comparison with economic interests, globalisation excludes a large part of the world's population. While some recent research attests to the benefits of globalisation, stating that per-capita global income more than tripled in the second half of the last century and that the indicators of human well-being improved as per-capita incomes rose (Sachs 2005), there is ample evidence that inequalities and gaps within countries and among countries grew.

According to the 2001 economics Nobel Prize winner Joseph Stiglitz (2003), globalisation has the potential to benefit humankind and is here to stay, but he also raises the question as to where we are going wrong. According to his analysis, free markets are good, but rich countries combine free markets with an important role for governments. Markets are the engine of the economy, but markets by themselves do not deliver benefits. Reforms, which the International Monetary Fund (IMF) and the World Bank demanded of poor countries as conditions for restructuring and dealing with growing debt burdens, were prerequisites, but carried out in the wrong way with the wrong pacing and the wrong sequencing.

Public spending on health, education and other social projects were cut, jobs were lost and poor countries and poor people became even poorer. The conditions demanded by the international financial institutions (IMF and the World Bank) for debt restructuring were drastic cuts in social spending, termed 'structural adjustment'. Healthcare and education suffered most. In addition to steep debt repayment schedules, poor countries lost their vital markets, because of agricultural subsidies and trade barriers in the North.

When facing the new global challenges, rich countries already had social institutions and safety nets in place, such as free universal education, universal healthcare, unemployment insurance and pension systems. They already had developed government regulations, including the legal systems for assuring sound economic transactions and accounting, while little of this existed in poor, developing countries and transition economies. Inequities in information and in understanding complex global economic processes added to widening the gap between rich and poor countries (Stiglitz 2003).

The net effect of the debt and reforms was an increase in stress and poverty within societies, leading to increased crime and urban violence. As societies in which there is a high level of violence are not attractive for investment, ignoring social concerns turned out not even to be good economic policy.

GLOBALISATION AND THE SOCIAL DETERMINANTS OF HEALTH

In a comprehensive review of globalisation and social determinants of health, Ronald Labonte and Ted Schrecker (2006) document and analyse the negative impact of globalisation on the well-being of people in developing and transition countries. They quote a large volume of research documenting growing poverty. All weak population groups suffer. While the research literature mentions in particular the effects on poor people, women and children, much anecdotal data attests to the negative effects on older people as well. This is particularly true in countries with a high HIV/AIDS burden, where older people, especially older women, care for their dying adult children and then are left to care for the orphans without the social or economic means to sustain themselves or their surviving grandchildren.

While some people have benefited from globalisation, most notably where public education and healthcare are well developed, the majority of poor people have no such benefits. Free trade, economic restructuring, the globalisation of finance, and the surge in migration, have in most parts of the world tended to produce harmful consequences. These developments have been overseen, and sometimes dictated, by inter-governmental organisations (IGOs) such as the IMF, the World Bank and the World Trade Organization (WTO), while other IGOs with less power have been limited to raising feeble warnings and protest.

GLOBALISATION AND FAMILIES

In the shift to globalisation, responsibility for health and social care and education was transferred from the governments of poor countries to families at the same time as families were losing their capacity to shoulder this responsibility. Opportunities for male employment and profit from traditional enterprises declined sharply in the South. In order to help their families survive, women tend to migrate, and the burden of globalisation is therefore largely shouldered by poor women. Entire communities live on remittances of migrants, but children and older people often suffer a vacuum of care. They are left behind by the women who migrate to rich countries in order to help their families to survive. Many of these caregivers become the carers of older persons in rich countries, while their own dependent children and elderly people are cared for by even poorer women, often from rural areas. Older women in rural areas then need to fill the gap and shoulder the caregiving work for small children and for sick and disabled persons left behind, while they themselves remain without the care they often need (Sassen 2002).

GLOBALISATION AND HEALTH

Global flows of money and information with direct impact on health involve people and their lifestyles as defined by consumption patterns. The 'communicability' of smoking and the associated burden of chronic diseases across national borders, by way of trade liberalisation and aggressive global tobacco marketing, is well known and documented (Bettcher *et al.* 2001; Pan American Health Organization (PAHO) 2003). Less familiar are the contributions of trade liberalisation and increased foreign direct investment in food processing and retailing to rapid increases in obesity in the developing world (Hawkes 2005; Ezzati *et al.* 2005).

These global developments have added considerably to the burden of chronic disease in developing countries. Tobacco is projected to be responsible for 10% of all deaths globally, killing 50% more people in 2015 than HIV/AIDS; and, in around one-third of people suffering from cardiovascular disease, the leading cause of death is linked to unbalanced nutrition, as are up to 30–40% of certain cancers (Mathers & Loncar 2006). One extreme example is that 88% of Micronesia's adult population is overweight (Brownell & Yach 2006). The impact of early death and disability on the economies of developing and transitional countries is immense. It is estimated China alone will lose over USD550 billion from lost productivity between 2005 and 2015, owing to chronic disease (WHO 2006a).

A more indirect effects of globalisation is large-scale urbanisation. Low crop prices and declining fertility mean that land ownership is a rapidly dwindling resource for older farmers, who struggle as their children leave the rural areas in search of waged labour (van Dullemen 2006). In reviewing the impact on the environment, Labonte & Schrecker (2006) cite numerous studies on the effects of urbanisation: exposure to vehicle traffic and air and water pollution, global migration of hazardous industries and waste, a lack of urban services, such as public transportation and affordable decent housing with safe water and sanitation, make life in large cities hazardous for urban poor people. The unprecedented scale of recent human impact on the natural environment, as in the case of global climate change (Haines *et al.* 2006), is one important health-related dimension in itself. Weak population groups, such as poor women, children and old people, are seriously affected by these processes.

A review of 76 studies specific to the health consequences of structural adjustment found a predominance of negative effects, highlighting that most studies found negative health impacts from structural adjustment in Africa (Breman & Shelton 2001). However, there are also serious consequences in other parts of the world. For instance, a national survey in Korea by Kim *et al.* (2003) found substantial increases in morbidity and decreases in health service utilisation following the 1997 currency crisis.

David Woodward *et al.* (2001) devised a model for focusing on five key linkages from globalisation to health. Direct effects include impacts on health systems, health policies, and exposure to certain hazards, such as infectious disease and tobacco marketing; indirect effects are the decreasing availability of resources for public expenditure on health, and on population risks, resulting from the impact of declining household income on nutrition and living conditions. There is no question that lack of resources is a major barrier to providing quality health services and to improving global health.

Laurie Garrett (2007), however, argues that improving global health cannot be achieved by the current strategies of putting nations on a USD20 billion charity programme and addressing selected health problems like HIV/AIDS, malaria or tuberculosis separately. The challenge remains of how to build not only effective national health systems and health infrastructures, but also local industries and franchises that can sustain health spending and thrive with increased health-related spending. Once international support wanes, local institutions will have to be ready to finance and provide sustainable health services in the longer run. One major challenge to improving health services globally is the growing crisis in the global health workforce.

GLOBALISATION AND HUMAN RESOURCES FOR HEALTH

The World Health Report 2006 *Working Together for Health* (WHO 2006b) analyses the current crisis in the global health workforce and presents proposals to tackle it over the next ten years. The report reveals an estimated shortage of almost 4.3 million doctors, midwives, nurses and support workers worldwide. The shortage is most severe in the poorest countries, especially in sub-Saharan Africa, where health workers are most needed.

Workers in health systems around the world, and nurses in particular, are experiencing increasing demands, stress and insecurity. Demographic and epidemiological transitions drive changes in population-based health threats to which the workforce must respond. Financing policies, technological advances and consumer expectations dramatically shift demands on the workforce in health systems. Concomitantly, health workers often face lack of job security in labour markets that are part of the global economy. In poor countries many workers face additionally demoralising working environments, such as poverty-level wages, unsupportive management, insufficient social recognition and weak career development. Despite these hardships, many health workers try their very best to provide decent care, but no matter how motivated and skilled health workers are, they cannot do their jobs properly in facilities that lack clean water, adequate lighting, heating, refrigeration, vehicles, drugs, working equipment and other essential supplies.

The spreading HIV/AIDS and tuberculosis epidemics impose huge work burdens, risks and threats. Additional demands derive from a growing number of people with multiple chronic diseases and a rapidly ageing population, often needing complex care. In many countries, health-sector reform under structural adjustment capped public-sector employment and limited investment in health worker education, thus drying up the supply of young graduates. Expanding labour markets have intensified professional concentration in urban areas and accelerated international migration from the poorest to the wealthiest countries. The consequent workforce crisis in many of the poorest countries is characterised by severe shortages, inappropriate skill mixes and gaps in service coverage (WHO 2006b).

The migration of skilled health workers is part of the growing global integrating of healthcare markets. The main destinations are the Gulf States, Europe and North America, where demand is increasing as national populations age. China has entered the market as a supplier of nurses; and, owing to political changes, such as the expansion of the European Union (EU), there is substantial movement of health professionals from the Czech Republic and Poland to the West, for example. Japan has also become a recipient country for health workers. Most migration follows broad former colonial, geographical and linguistic ties (Connell & Stilwell 2006; Maybud & Wiskow 2006).

The exodus of health professionals has jeopardised health services in many of the poorest source countries. In 2002, the vacancy rate for doctors in Ghana was 47.3% and the rate of unfilled posts for registered nurses was 57%. Malawi reported a 52% vacancy rate for nurses. While South Africa is losing health workers to richer countries, it recruits from abroad to fill its own shortage. In 1999, 78% of rural doctors were non-South Africans, coming mainly from Kenya, Malawi and Zimbabwe. Recruitment agencies play an important role in this global healthcare market. Their activities range from recruiting healthcare professionals from Cameroon to marketing Polish doctors in the United Kingdom, to recruiting Fijian nurses for the United Arab Emirates (UAE) and New Zealand. These agencies invest considerable funds in this lucrative business (Maybud & Wiskow 2006; Connell & Stilwell 2006).

The WHO (2006b) estimates that there are currently 57 countries with critical shortages, equivalent to a global deficit of 2.4 million doctors, nurses and midwives. The proportional shortfalls are greatest in sub-Saharan Africa, although numerical deficits are very large in Southeast Asia because of its population size. Paradoxically, these shortages often coexist in countries with large numbers of unemployed health professionals. Poverty, lack of public funds and bureaucratic red tape, among other causes, produce this paradox of shortages in the midst of underutilised human capital. Ethical recruitment becomes a major concern.

Almost all countries suffer from maldistribution of the workforce, characterised by urban concentration and rural deficits, but these imbalances are perhaps most disturbing when considering the role of international migration. The huge nursing shortage projected for countries such as the US (nearly half a million by the year 2015) and Canada (113 000 by 2011) is serving as a magnet for nurses with a command of English, thus adversely affecting other countries. In the Caribbean, an average of 35% of nursing positions are unfilled, despite the traditional excellence in nursing education; in Jamaica and Trinidad and Tobago, the figure has reached 50%. The nursing brain drain is also being felt in South America.

Peru's national nursing association reported that between 2002 and 2006 more than 5000 nurses, or 15% of the nursing workforce, have emigrated, primarily to Spain, Italy and the US (PAHO 2005; PAHO 2006).

The overall scale of the shortages is staggering. It is estimated that sub-Saharan Africa has a shortfall of more than 600 000 nurses in relation to the numbers required for scaling up priority interventions, as recommended by the Commission on Macroeconomics and Health. Many European countries also report nursing shortages. Australia projects a shortage of 40 000 by 2010 (Buchan & Calman 2004). The US Department of Health and Human Services estimates that the shortage of nurses in the US will grow to 275 000 by 2010 and to 800 000 by 2020. Eleven per cent of the US registered nurse workforce (303 000 nurses) were 'foreign born' and, of these, 70% immigrated from developing countries. In quoting these figures, Linda Aiken (2006) states that the future of the global nursing shortage will largely depend on the US and other wealthy countries' efforts to become far more self-sufficient in relation to their health workforce. At present, American nursing schools reject more than 150 000 qualified applicants every year, owing to the lack of nursing faculty. Yet every year the US Congress has refused to pass bills augmenting nursing professors' salaries, while sponsoring legislation eliminating all caps on immigration of foreign nurses. In 2005 alone, Congress set aside 50 000 special immigration visas for nurses (Garrett 2007).

The nursing shortage in rich countries also accelerates the physician shortages in poor countries. Since the year 2000, more than 3500 Filipino physicians have taken accelerated nursing courses and have left for jobs abroad. More than 4000 physicians (internists, surgeons, anaesthesiologists, family practitioners and sub-specialists) are now in nursing school in the Philippines (Domingo & Salvana 2006). More than one quarter of the overall physician workforce in Australia, Canada, the UK and the US are immigrants, with 40% (Australia) and 75% (UK) of them coming from lower-income countries (Mullan 2005).

While 'active' recruitment by wealthy countries is decried as unethical, as it deprives the health systems of poor countries of vital human capital, health worker migration must be understood in the broader context of global labour movements. Often as important as international flows is migration from rural to urban areas, from public-sector to private-sector employment, or from nursing (health sector) to non-nursing, or no employment. While there is no doubt that ethical recruitment and compensation to poor countries need to be seriously considered, nurses (and physicians) often exercise the right to move, as they cannot exercise the right to stay (Buchan & Calman 2004) if they want academic opportunities and the chance to support their families and offer their children a good education and a better future.

However, the implications of the brain drain are serious. Poor regions and countries lose vital human resources. Many of these countries are dealing simultaneously with infectious diseases and the rapid emergence of chronic illnesses complicated by the magnitude of the HIV/AIDS epidemic. All care, and in particular the availability of vaccines and drugs to cope with these health threats, requires a sophisticated workforce (doctors, nurses, laboratory workers, managerial staff and others) in sufficient numbers, with the right geographic distribution in health facilities providing universal coverage.

Developing and sustaining a long-term care labour force is particularly challenging, as long-term care (LTC) relies heavily on human labour. While the bulk of care is provided by families worldwide, there is a need for a large cadre of people providing care in disparate locations, seven days a week, 24 hours a day. LTC work has less prestige than hospital work for health professionals, and the frontline workers (personal care workers, aides, home health aids, home health attendants, home care workers) have even less prestige. Working conditions are poor and there are usually no career prospects (Kane 2003; *Canadian Home Care Human Resources Study* 2003).

In the US, paid dependency work is largely carried out by women of colour, and among men, disproportionately by men of colour. Migrant women, primarily from poor countries, provide this essential service, leaving their own dependent children and old relatives lacking care. Eva Feder Kittay *et al.* (2005) and Sadkia Sassen (2002) describe not only the mechanisms underlying these global trends, but also the dire ethical implications. The burden of care in rich countries is now shouldered by poor women who enable the survival of their families in a global environment, by 'love's labour'. The work is physically and emotionally demanding and the working conditions are usually very poor, with long working hours, few social benefits and poor pay.

DEVELOPING A GLOBAL NURSING ETHIC

The essence of a global ethic is based on the knowledge of what it means to be a human being, despite cultural, religious, ethnic, political, gender, age and economic differences. I have chosen Amartya Sen's (in Nussbaum 2002) human capabilities as the benchmark on which to base the development of a global nursing ethic. Sen has identified 10 central human capabilities that have a direct link to our central nursing responsibilities or functions.* While not

---

* 'The unique function of the nurse is to assist the individual, sick or well, in the performance of those activities contributing to health or its recovery (or to a peaceful death) that he would perform unaided if he had the necessary strength, will or knowledge. And to do this in such a way as to help him gain independence, as rapidly as possible.'(Henderson 1966) While this definition needs to be expanded to describe also the function of nursing in regard to families, communities, aggregates and health policy, its nucleus is still valid.

all these capabilities are the primary responsibility of nursing, they all need to be considered in the care we provide, as well as in the concern for the nursing workforce.

CENTRAL HUMAN CAPABILITIES

Life: To be able to live to the end of a human life of normal length; not dying prematurely, or before one's life is so reduced as to be not worth living.

Bodily health: Able to have good health, including nourishment and shelter.

Bodily integrity: Being able to move freely from place to place; to be secure against assault.

Senses, imagination, and thought: Being able to imagine, think and reason in a truly 'human' way, informed and cultivated by education and the arts; protected by guarantees of freedom of expression.

Emotions: Being able to love those who love and care for us, to grieve at their absence; to experience longing, love, gratitude and justified anger; not having one's emotional development blighted by fear and anxiety.

Practical reason: Being able to form a conception of the good and to engage in critical reflection about the planning of one's life.

Affiliation: Being able to live with others, to recognise and show concern for other human beings, to engage in social interaction, to be able to imagine the situation of another. (This includes protecting freedom of assembly and political and religious freedoms.)

Other species: Being able to live with concern for and in relation to animals, plants and the world of nature.

Play: Being able to laugh, to play, to enjoy recreational activities.

Control over one's environment: Politically, being able to participate effectively in political choices that govern one's life; materially, having property rights and the right to seek employment on an equal basis with others; in work, being able to work as a human being, with meaningful relationships of mutual recognition with other workers.

It will take much collaborative work of nurse ethicists around the globe to develop a genuine global nursing ethic. This will require much thought and discussions on how these and other theoretical conceptions can be moulded into a coherent system that can help to explain complex situations and guide nurses in their practice. It also requires much 'bottom-up' work, where the thinking and dilemmas of nurses in their daily practice in hospitals and in the communities are analysed. This bottom-up qualitative research on which to base a nursing ethic will have to represent a wide range of cultural, religious, ethnic, political, gender, age and economic nursing experience. This requires nurse researchers and ethicists from all the world's sub-regions to develop a common understanding of the crucial issues to be explored; and then to develop a shared research protocol.

This is one area where we could demonstrate how globalisation is 'good'. Such a project could promote a better understanding and, hopefully, much better practice, thus benefiting nurses and those for whom we care. Without the global technology of the Internet and email communication, one could not even dream of such a project. Another vital link for such a project is access to the scientific literature for all nurses who would wish to participate, regardless of the country in which they live and regardless of the usual economic barriers. This dream has become real through the WHO Health InterNetwork Access to Research Initiative (HINARI), which provides free or very low-cost online access to the major journals in biomedical and related social sciences to local not-for-profit institutions in developing countries.*

THE CHALLENGE TO NURSING

When considering the topic 'Globalisation: good or bad, and for whom?', the matter of who shoulders responsibility is raised. While the vast majority of nurses have little influence and control over major economic and political developments (very few nurses are in political decision-making and leading economic positions), all nurses can make a difference in trying to tilt the balance from bad to good, or at least, to less negative.

This requires first and foremost that nurses realise it is no longer acceptable to be aware only of their own country's demographic, epidemiological, socio-economic and political changes; bacteria, viruses and trends impacting on health do not respect borders. At the very least national nursing leadership needs to understand and monitor global changes and try to understand their impact on local realities. Together with others, nurses need then to develop scenarios on how to make use of new opportunities and how best to forestall negative impact.

---

* Local, not-for-profit institutions in two groups of countries may register for access to the journals through HINARI. The country lists are based on GNP per capita (World Bank figures, 2001). Institutions in countries with GNP per capita below USD1000 are eligible for free access. Institutions in countries with GNP per capita of USD1000–3000 pay a fee of USD1000 per year per institution. Eligible categories of institutions are: national universities, research institutes, professional schools (medicine, nursing, pharmacy, public health, dentistry), teaching hospitals, government offices and national medical libraries. All staff members and students are entitled to access to the journals. For more information, see http://www.who.int/hinari/about/en/.

There is a need to develop new policies to guide health, education and welfare, all of which are crucial for nursing, and then to create the tools necessary to implement these policies. None of this is possible without the ability to create coalitions, develop regulatory systems and foster accountability.

While these tasks seem to be the major responsibility of a national and international nursing leadership, all nurses can and should provide the bottom-up intelligence to inform new policies. In order for this to be possible however, nurses need a sound basic education in epidemiology and social change, as well as monitoring tools and reporting systems that are easy to use. Providing bottom-up intelligence must also be seen as an integral part of nurses' responsibilities, with working conditions taking account of this complex task, for example, time allocated for training and sufficient staffing to address these and other tasks, as well as adequate pay.

In order to understand the full impact of globalisation, we will need to monitor the global debates and developments (political, economic, trade, health trends) constantly, as well as their impact on our local realities. This is a very demanding task. Its only chance to succeed even partially is for WHO, the International Council of Nurses (ICN), the International Council of Midwives (ICM), and other national and international nursing and health worker/professional organisations to accept this as a challenge. Universities and research centres worldwide will have to join in. In order to address such a challenge in an effective way, considerable efforts and resources will be required. Only with such a global commitment will nurses individually and nursing as a profession be able to participate effectively in the globalisation debate.

REFERENCES

Aiken LH. U.S. *Policies: Key to global nurse sufficiency.* 2006. Available at: http://www. academyhealth.org/NHPC/foreignpolicy/2006/aiken.ppt#608,11 (accessed 5 May 2007).

Bettcher D, Soll L, Subramanian C, Grabman G, Guindon E, Joossens L, Perucic A, Taylor A. *Confronting the Tobacco Epidemic in an Era of Trade Liberalization.* Report WG4: 9. Cambridge, MA: Commission on Macroeconomics and Health; 2001.

Breman A, Shelton C. *Structural Adjustment and Health: a literature review of the debate, its role-players and presented empirical evidence.* Report WG6: 6. Cambridge, MA: Commission on Macroeconomics and Health; 2001.

Brownell KD, Yach D. *Lessons from a Small Country About the Global Obesity Crisis.* 2006. Available at: http://www.globalizationandhealth.com/content/pdf/1744-8603-2-11.pdf (accessed 5 May 2007).

Buchan J, Calman L. *The Global Shortage of Registered Nurses: an overview of issues and actions.* 2004. Available at: http://www.icn.ch/global/shortage.pdf (accessed 5 May 2007).

Canadian Home Care Human Resources Study. 2003. Available at: http://www.cacc-acssc.com/ english/pdf/homecareresources/EngTechnic.pdf (accessed 5 May 2007).

Commission on Macroeconomics and Health. Available at: http://www.cmhealth.org/cmh_papers&reports.htm or http://www.who.int/macrohealth/en/ (accessed 17 May 2007).

Connell J, Stilwell B. Merchants of Medical Care: recruiting agencies in the global health chain. In: Kuptsch C, editor. *Merchants of Labour*. Geneva: International Institute for Labour Studies; 2006.

Domingo AF, Salvana EMT. Letter to the editor. *New England Journal of Medicine*. 2006; **354**(5): 529.

Encyclopedia Britannica. Volume 5, Micropedia. 15th ed. Jacob E Safra, Chairman of the Board. Ilan Yeshua, Chief Executive Officer. Chicago, IL: The New Encyclopedia Britannica Inc. 2002.

Ezzati M, Van der Hoorn S, Lawes CMM, *et al*. Rethinking the 'Diseases of Affluence' Paradigm: global patterns of nutritional risks in relation to economic development. PLoS *Medicine*. 2005; **2**(5): e133.

Feder Kittay E, Jennings B, Wassuna AA. Dependency, Difference and the Global Ethic of Long Term Care. *The Journal of Political Philosophy*. 2005; **13**(4): 443–69.

Garrett L. The Challenge of Global Health: beware what you wish for. *Foreign Affairs*. 2007; **86**(1): 14–38, 25.

Haines A, Kovats RS, Campbell-Lendrum D, Carvalan C. Climate Change and Human Health: impacts, vulnerability, and mitigation. *Lancet*. 2006; **367**: 2101–09.

Hawkes C. The Role of Foreign Direct Investment in the Nutrition Transition. *Public Health Nutrition*. 2005; **8**(4): 357–65.

Henderson V. *The Nature of Nursing: a definition and its implications for practice, research, and education*. New York: Macmillan; 1966.

Jenkins R. Globalization, Production, Employment and Poverty: debates and evidence. *Journal of International Development*. 2004; **16**: 1–12.

Kane RA. Human Resources for Long Term Care: lessons from the United States experience. In: Brodsky J, Habib J, Hirschfeld M, editors. *Key Policy Issues in Long-term Care*. Geneva: World Health Organization; 2003.

Kim H, Chung WJ, Song YJ, *et al*. Changes in Morbidity and Medical Care Utilization After the Recent Economic Crisis in the Republic of Korea. *Bulletin World Health Organization*. 2003; **81**(8): 567–72.

Labonte R, Schrecker T. 2006. *Globalization and Social Determinants of Health: analytic and strategic paper*. Available at: http://www.who.int/social_determinants/resources/globalization.pdf (accessed 5 May 2007).

Mathers CD, Loncar D. Projections of Global Mortality and Burden of Disease from 2002 to 2030. PLoS *Medicine*. 2006; **3**(11): e442. Available at: http://medicine.plosjournals.org/archive/1549-1676/3/11/pdf/10.1371_journal.pmed.0030442-L.pdf (accessed 5 May 2007).

Maybud S, Wiskow C. 'Care Trade': the international brokering of health care professionals. In: Kuptsch C, editor. *Merchants of Labour*. Geneva: International Institute for Labour Studies; 2006. Available at: http://www.ilo.org/public/english/bureau/inst/download/merchants.pdf (accessed 5 May 2007).

Mullan F. The Metrics of Physician Brain Drain. *New England Journal of Medicine*. 2005; **353**(17): 1810–18.

Nussbaum MC. Long-term Care and Social Justice: a challenge to conventional ideas of the social contract. Appendix A, pp. 31–65. In: *Ethical Choices in Long-term Care: what does justice require?* Geneva: World Health Organization; 2002.

PAHO. *Profits Over People: tobacco industry activities to market cigarettes and undermine public health in Latin America and the Caribbean*. Washington DC: PAHO; 2003.

PAHO. Nursing Shortage Threatens Health Care. Newsletter of PAHO. September 2005. Available at: http://www.paho.org/English/DD/PIN/ptoday18_sep05.htm (accessed 5 May 2007).

PAHO. 2006. *Everyday Heroes: health workers*. Message of the director of the PAHO, Dr Mirta Roses Periago. Available at: http://www.paho.org/English/D/WorldHealthDay-Eng-Apr7-06.htm (accessed 5 May 2007).

Sachs JD. *The End of Poverty*. London: Penguin; 2005.

Sassen S. Women's Burden: counter-geographies of globalization and the feminization of survival. *Nordic Journal of International Law*. 2002; **71**(2): 255–74.

Stiglitz JE. *Globalization and its Discontent*. New York: Norton; 2003.

van Dullemen, C. Older People in Africa: new engines to society? *National Women's Studies Association Journal*. 2006; **18**(1): 99–105.

WHO. WPR/RC57/6 report on progress. Western Pacific Regional Office (WPRO) Regional Committee Meeting, Auckland, New Zealand, 18–22 September, 2006a.

WHO. *Working Together for Health*. The World Health Report 2006. Geneva: World Health Organization; 2006b. Available at: http://www.who.int/whr/2006/en/index.html (accessed 5 May 2007).

Woodward D, Drager N, Beaglehole R, Lipson D. *Globalization and Health: a framework for analysis and action*. Report WG4: 10. Cambridge, MA: Commission on Macroeconomics and Health; 2001.

Values, rights and responsibilities

3

On being ethical in a global community: what is a nurse to do?

Wendy Austin

INTRODUCTION

Thomas Nagel (1986, p. 12) acknowledges that 'I do not feel equal to the problems treated in this book'. I want to make a similar disclaimer here: I do not feel equal to the question of what an individual nurse may do to practise ethically in our contemporary world. Rather, it is a question with which I struggle and have been struggling for some time. I believe that the best way for me to contribute to its exploration by others is to describe my personal efforts with it, to identify some of the more troublesome aspects of my search for an answer, and to share my thoughts on a way for the individual nurse to understand, consider and act on professional responsibilities within a global community.

About six years ago, I had the privilege to teach for a term at the University of Ghana. While in Ghana I wrote an article in which I asked, 'What changes for nursing ethics when the global, not the local, becomes the dominant frame of reference?' (Austin 2001). The article was a way of working through a shift in thinking that had been happening for me. Just previously, I had been on a research fellowship studying health ethics while concurrently working with my faculty to achieve designation as a WHO Collaborating Centre in nursing and mental health. Throughout this period of about two years, a significant change occurred for me and for those with whom I was working and learning: 'international' bioethics became 'global' health ethics. It was rather suddenly, it seemed, less about sharing national perspectives on ethics and more about understanding that a process of globalisation was occurring, *had* occurred, and that the global village predicted by Marshall McLuhan (1964), or some form of it, was at hand. The greatest threats to our survival as individuals and communities were not domestic in scope, but rather global: the effects of human activities on the environment, nuclear weaponry, emerging and resurgent infectious diseases, chemical and biological terrorism (Jowitt 1992) and, for nearly half of us, devastating poverty. Our moral space was being redefined and it seemed that the Nobel Laureate, Oscar Arias Sanchez, was right when he warned that the twenty-first century cannot survive with the ethics of the twentieth century (Sanchez 1997).

AIMING FOR AN ETHICAL LIFE

Paul Ricouer (1992, p. 192) has defined ethics as 'aiming at the "good life" with and for others in just institutions'. How do we aim for this good life within the contemporary global community? How should we understand our rights, duties and responsibilities to one another? If I take seriously the idea that everyone, regardless of their economic and geographic situation, has a right to the opportunity for a healthy life, how should I, as a nurse, act? What should I do?

I began the article I wrote in Ghana with an image of our planet. When we travelled to space and saw Earth for the first time, we could see ourselves as we truly are, dwelling together, on a finite globe, turning slowly through space. What happens on our planet, not just environmental events, but economic, political and military ones, are global events. The boundaries on our maps are illusions. Earth itself is a living entity. James Lovelock's (1979) Gaia theory – developed when he was assigned by the National Aeronautics and Space Administration (NASA) to consider the possibility of life on Mars, which lead him to consider life on Earth more deeply – suggests convincingly that our planet is a self-regulating, interconnected system based more on cooperation than on competition.

The technological prowess that took us to space changed, and continues to change, the very nature of our day-to-day existence. Several years ago, one of Canada's Aboriginal elders, Chief Dan George (1975, p. 16) wrote an open letter he entitled, 'I was born 1000 years ago . . .' Born in 1899, he describes being born into a culture of bows and arrows, and being flung across the ages to the culture of the atom bomb. He wrote '. . . and from bows and arrows to atom bombs is a distance far beyond the flight to the moon.'

Paradoxically, as people are coming together, we are also being driven further apart (Bauman 1998). Economic globalisation is fostering a hegemonic view of the world as a marketplace (Freidman 1999), where the value of a person is based on the capacity to be a consumer. Chief Dan George described how his people did not have the time to take twentieth-century progress and eat it little by little, and digest it. They did not have the skills to make a meaningful contribution to this kind of world. This made them lose pride in themselves as a people and as individuals. They live now in a world where the wisdom of a Chief Dan George is not authentically valued.

Globalisation is fostering an incredible chasm between the technologically connected and those not connected, between people who are rich and people who are poor, with the latter being separated and excluded. At the beginning of the twentieth century, when Chief Dan George was born, the disparity between the top 20% and the bottom 20% of the world's population was a ninefold difference. It was 80-fold by the year 2000 and continues to grow (Benatar *et al.* 2005). The global village is not becoming as some imagined, a place in which life chances become equitable for all. Health for all, which we had envisioned as a reality by the end of the twentieth century, still eludes us, despite our scientific achievements.

When I returned home from Ghana, it was to the good news that a member of my family, Ivy, had had a successful lung transplant. I was amazed to be with Ivy in a restaurant three weeks after her surgery: she was vibrant and full of plans. She only lived a further 10 months, owing to a return of cancer, perhaps the effect of her immunosuppressant drugs. Those months mattered much to her family, and Ivy was there for the birth of two new grandchildren. How different our story was from that of the families I had met in Ghana; how different our healthcare resources.

When in Ghana, I taught an advanced clinical course that included caring for persons with HIV/AIDS. The patients with AIDS had no access to antiviral medications, and often could not afford adequate food or other critical things, such as schooling for their children. I floundered, trying to find a way to think about the great disparities between opportunities for a healthy life. How could it be ethical for these to continue to exist?

I wrote another article (the coping device of academics?), now a chapter in the book edited by Jan Storch and colleagues, *Toward a Moral Horizon* (Austin 2004). In that chapter, I described being confronted in a personal and close-up way with the inequalities of our global community, and called for nurses to be attentive to what was happening outside their immediate geographical community. I quoted Michael Ignatieff (1997), that our moral space can no longer be divided readily into those for whom we have responsibility and those we do not.

MY RESPONSIBILITIES AS A NURSE

The International Council of Nurses (ICN) *Code of Ethics for Nurses* (ICN, 2006) stipulates that, as a nurse, I share with others and with society as a whole a *responsibility* for action that meets the health and social needs of the public, especially its most vulnerable members. I agree strongly with the code. I described the ways in which nurses can be responsible in a global community and can address some of the barriers to achieving health for all:

- ❑ by ethical attentiveness
- ❑ use a primary healthcare approach
- ❑ be informed
- ❑ raise the consciousness of others
- ❑ get professional associations involved
- ❑ influence the political climate: make it safe to speak (Austin 2004).

I had, nevertheless, a nagging sense of not truly meeting my responsibilities, of failing what I was encouraging others to do. Zygmunt Bauman (1993, p. 242) has it right when he calls it: 'cumbersome, incapacitating, joy-killing, insomniogenic moral responsibility'.

My work with our WHO Collaborating Centre was allowing me to see health disparities close-up in parts of the world other than Africa: for example, the 100-year-old mental hospital in St Lucia, where very few nurses were trying to care for around 150 patients, and where the 56 female patients slept in one room, and the male patients' main recreation was watching cruise ships (as tall as skyscrapers) dock. Though we were trying to contribute to reform, it seemed to me that we were not accomplishing much. I found it very frustrating and distressing. I was somewhat – shamefully – relieved when a research chair took me away from this work.

MORAL DISTRESS

My research is focused on relational ethics, an approach that makes explicit that ethics needs to be about more than moral reasoning. It moves us to raise questions often not addressed in traditional bioethics. A study in relational ethics in mental healthcare led us to explore mental health practitioners' experience of moral distress. Moral distress is not an everyday term. I like this definition (Nathaniel 2002, p. 5): 'It is the pain or anguish affecting the mind, body or relationships in response to a situation in which the person is aware of a moral problem, acknowledges moral responsibility, and makes a moral judgement about the correct action; yet, as a result of real or perceived constraints, participates in perceived moral wrongdoing.'

Moral distress affects how one feels about one's self and one's integrity. Albert Camus (1957) elegantly portrays this in his novel, *The Fall*. In this novel, the narrator tells a stranger in a bar in Amsterdam about his past as an enviable Parisian lawyer who 'was truly above reproach in [his] professional life'. He tells the stranger (p. 20): 'I enjoyed my own nature to the fullest, and we all know that there lies happiness.' One momentous night, however, as he is returning home after midnight by way of the Pont Royal, he passes a young woman staring at the river. He is about 50 yards away when he hears a sound of a body striking water. He stops but does not turn around; he hears a cry, repeated many times, fading, and then no more. He describes wanting to run but an irresistible weakness comes over him; slowly he walks away. From this time on, his life and his sense of himself is changed. He dreams nightly of having a second chance to save both the woman and himself.

Like Camus' character, health practitioners can experience lasting effects from morally distressing situations in which they fail to live up to their own expectations of themselves. Unfortunately, this can happen even when the constraints on moral action are external ones. For example, a Canadian, Lieutenant-General Romeo Dallaire, was in charge of the UN peacekeeping force in Rwanda in the early 1990s. He was unable to get the necessary permission and support to prevent the massacre of hundreds of thousands of Rwandans. In his book, *Shake Hands with the Devil* (Dallaire 2003), he tells of his belief in his and our moral responsibility to the people of Rwanda. He reveals his extreme distress at being unable to carry out his mission and to respond in the way he believed that, as a military commander and as a person, he ought. (Now Senator Dallaire, he is trying with little success to get Canada to play a more effective role in stopping the genocide in Darfur.)

For moral distress to occur, a person must be aware of a moral problem and acknowledge moral responsibility. I began to wonder if, by pointing to the terrible disparities in global health and naming nurses' responsibilities, I was not provoking moral distress. One morning at a symposium at our ethics centre, after my presentation on health practitioners' responsibility in global health, I was told that I was. A young man raised his hand and said: 'Wendy, my morale was really low when I came here today. I am really unhappy with the way time constraints on care-giving and a narrow focus on cost are affecting my practice. And now you make me feel worse.' Although he nodded in understanding when I responded that the same forces shaping his local practice were those contributing to, even causing, the global health problems I identified, there was a moment of troubled silence when I simply stared at him and was without words of comfort or inspiration.

What do I mean when I argue that this young man and I have a responsibility, as nurses, to everyone on Earth? Said in this way, it seems rather ludicrous. Yet there seems an essential truth to it. How do we enact such a terrifying responsibility? I needed to take a step back and think about responsibility itself, to consider how much of what happens in the world *belongs* to me and *puts claims* on me (Rorty 1999).

THINKING ABOUT RESPONSIBILITY

It is a universal principle that not *harming others* is basic to an ethical life. It seems so obvious that students expect to skim over it in ethics classes. (I always think of an old H*agar the Horrible* cartoon in which Hagar's physician tries to reassure him with: 'Don't worry. The doctors' motto is "do no harm".' When the physician leaves, Hagar's wife, Helga, asks him, 'Doesn't it worry you that they have to *think* of that?'). We know, however, that this basic rule of responsibility is not so simple, and most moral philosophers believe that our responsibility to one another goes far beyond not harming.

Arthur Schopenhauer's (1965, p. 65) motto for ethics is: 'Harm no one, on the contrary, help as many people as you can.' We need to be compassionate. Compassion, according to Schopenhauer, means to see the suffering of others and want to do something about it. In Confucian ethics the symbol (JEN) for compassion (also translated as humaneness) is composed of the symbols for person and for two (Yutang 1943). It captures Emmanuel Levinas' idea of our responsibility or 'responsivity' to one another (Levinas 1987, p. 21). Whenever there are two, the face of the other calls to us. Ethics is lived in our response to the other before us. When the other is faceless, as in a crowd, atrocities like genocide can happen.

Albert Schweitzer believed that ethics is nothing else than reverence for life. When life is sacred to us (the lives of plants and animals as well as those of fellow humans), we act helpfully to all life that is in need. Ethics, says Schweitzer (1946, p. 311) is 'responsibility without limit towards all that lives'. A contemporary philosopher, Raimond Gaita (2000, p. 15), believes that someone who affirms the preciousness of every human being will act differently than someone who cannot or will not do so. For him, our morality is affected by whether or not we find, as he puts it, the conceptual space to see one another. It matters if we are invisible or only partly visible to one another.

These ethicists, whose work I find compelling, demand more than doing no harm for living an ethical life. They expect the ethical person to be able to *see* when another is suffering, and to respond. They recognise that they are making a profound claim. Levinas (1987, p. 22) said, 'Ethics is the experience of a demand that we both cannot fully meet and cannot avoid.' Schweitzer (1946, p. 254) wrote, 'The ethics of reverence for life throws upon us a responsibility so unlimited as to be terrifying.'

One way we try to deal with such *terrifying* responsibility to others has been to limit who the others might be. For instance, we may limit the scope of our obligations to our own family or, as a nurse, to the patients directly in front of us. Ethicists call this the principle of proximity. We may limit our zone of responsibility to fellow citizens of our political community or geographic area. For example, John Rawls' (1973) work on obligations of justice, on the whole, assumed a single, relatively closed community, although his *The Law of Peoples* (1999) does apply across societies.

Nevertheless, this delimiting of responsibility has been challenged at least since biblical times. The parable of the Good Samaritan (Holy Bible) relates how a man from Jerusalem is set upon by thieves and left for dead. It is a stranger, a Samaritan, who shows him compassion and comes to his aid. In this action, the Samaritan is revealed as a true neighbour. But can we be true neighbours to everyone in our global community?

This question is raised through a different analogy, offered by Richard Rorty at a United Nations Educational, Scientific and Cultural Organization (UNESCO) gathering that examined the question: Who are the members of our moral community? Rorty (1996) uses the analogy of triage to suggest that it may not be feasible to include everyone on Earth as members of our moral community. A willingness to help all is not enough; there needs to be the belief that one can actually help them. He argues:

> When we realize that it is unfeasible to rescue a person or a group, it is as if they had already gone before us into death. Such people are, as we say, "dead to us".... For the sake of their own sanity, and for the sake of the less grievously wounded patients who *are* admitted to the hospital, the doctors and nurses must simply blank out on all those moaning victims who are left outside in the street. They must cease to think about them, pretend they are already dead. These doctors and nurses illustrate the point that if you cannot render assistance to people in need, your claim that they form part of your moral community is empty (p. 13).

This triage analogy is not helpful to me in trying to work out how to enact my responsibility as a nurse in a global village. Primarily, because as I nurse I know we are *not* in a triage situation. We have the means – the knowledge and the wealth – to bring health to all. Stephen Lewis, the UN Secretary-General's special envoy on HIV/AIDS in Africa, writes in his book *Race Against Time* (Lewis 2005, p. 166), 'between daily misery on one hand, and well-being on the other, there stands only the decision by the rich nations to share a tiny fraction of their wealth'. Lewis argues that, despite laudatory efforts by WHO and UNAIDS, we are losing the race against time because the money committed to fight HIV/ AIDS, as well as tuberculosis (TB) and malaria, is inadequate. Although the G8 countries, among others, made a promise 37 years ago to give 0.7% of their GNP to foreign aid (Lewis, 2005, p. 149), none of them have. When they do give aid, much of it can be termed 'phantom aid'. Jeffrey Sachs in *The End of Poverty* (2005) describes how, of the USD3 in aid the US gave for every sub-Saharan African in 2002, the amount actually received was six cents, once the amounts for US technical consultants, for food and emergency aid, administrative costs and debt relief are taken into account.

Triage might have been a helpful model for nurses to use to prioritise their responsibilities in a global community; it is one we know and use. However, not only are we not in a triage situation, but the principles of triage are not being followed when it comes to global health. Triage decisions are based on saving the most lives with the resources one has. Even as we plan for a predicted pandemic – a public health emergency in which the good of the community clearly trumps the good of the individual – we are not using principles of triage. In North America and Europe at least, there seems to be a media frenzy about avian flu (H5N1), which has killed fewer than 200 people (WHO 2007). Where is the frenzy over malaria? Three thousand children die every day of malaria. It kills in a month as many as died in the 2004 Tsunami. TB infects nine million people a year and kills two million. HIV/AIDS kills three million. We should be able to say, as does the narrator at the end of Camus' novel *The Plague*: 'From now on it can be said that the plague was the concern of all of us' (Camus 1947, p. 57), but we cannot. The triage model, despite its possibilities for helping nurses to conceptualise their responsibilities, cannot be realised, given the current context of the global village.

There is another rather famous contemporary moral paradigm regarding responsibility: that of a child drowning in a pond. Peter Singer uses it to question why, if it is morally reprehensible to pass by a child drowning in a pond when one could save her, 'I was late' or 'I didn't want to get the cuffs of my pants wet' will not be an acceptable excuses to anyone. It is not just as morally reprehensible to fail to put a cheque in an envelope and send it to where it can save a starving child (1972, p. 6). The latter may take even less effort.

Singer, and others such as Peter Unger, author of *Living High and Letting Die* (1996), share a model of ethical responsibility, termed by some as a cosmopolitan utilitarian model, in which the moral imperative is to decrease suffering. They argue that giving up one's luxuries in order to help others who are suffering is essential to the ethical life. Affluent people and societies should give what they can and whatever is surplus to their needs. It is the decent thing to do.

There are those who strongly disagree with this model of responsibility. Neera Badhwar, in an article in *Social Philosophy & Policy Foundation* (2006, p. 73) says this view 'clashes with common sense' and that 'If Singer and Unger are right about what is required for moral decency, or even for the ideally moral life, then practically no one is morally decent.' Acting as they suggest, she argues, would mean giving up the prospect of happiness (p. 86), and that is incompatible with that which makes life worth living. For her, such a take on moral responsibility denies our entitlement to use our time and resources in ways that we find meaningful and enjoyable, and thus denies our integrity. Her response to Singer's drowning child is stark:

> Just as children die every day from absolute poverty in distant lands, we might say so children die every day from drowning in front of our eyes. A terrible thing, yes, but what can one do? We all have our own lives to lead: we can at best save a few from drowning every year; it's the system that leads to drowning children that needs to be fixed (Badhwar 2006, p. 81).

She agrees that the system needs fixing, but not by aid: 'Even if activities of aid were beneficial . . . if most of us gave away all our "spare" money instead of investing it in worthwhile enterprises or spending it on "luxuries" we would push even more people into the ranks of the absolutely poor.' She asks, 'if we came across someone drowning or bleeding to death every time we stepped out, how long would we continue to be good Samaritans?' (Badhwar 2006, p. 81). How can anyone argue that we should sacrifice all our aspirations and projects to the task of saving people?

Thomas Pogge (2005), author of *World Poverty and Human Rights*, sees the 'drowning child in a pond' differently from both Singer and Badhwar. He argues that we have pushed the child into the pond. At the very least, it is our responsibility to stop doing that. The do-no-harm approach to responsibility alone will do wonders if we stop shaping and enforcing the social conditions that, foreseeably and avoidably, cause the monumental suffering of the poor. Pogge (2005, p. 33) is very strong on this: we must stop being active participants in a crime against humanity. He protests that 'Hitler and Stalin were vastly more evil than our political leaders, but in terms of killing and harming people they never came anywhere near causing 18 million deaths per year.'

With less passion but along the same lines, Robert Goodin (1985), in *Protecting the Vulnerable*, develops a 'vulnerability model' of ethical responsibility. His principle is that 'we are responsible for protecting those vulnerable to our actions and choices' and 'Our responsibilities to persons are proportional to the degree to which they are dependent upon you (and you alone) to perform certain services and to the degree with which your actions and choices affect their interests.' (p. 117) His ideas of responsibility are in many respects congruent to that of feminist ethicists, such as Onora O'Neill (1985) and Margaret Walker (1998).

A SOCIAL CONNECTION MODEL OF RESPONSIBILITY

Recently, a new social connection model has been articulated by Iris Young (2006), a sociologist. She asks how we will conceptualise responsibility for structural injustice. In her answer, she stipulates that people have responsibility by virtue of their social roles (nurse, professor, citizen). Her social connection model is forward looking: individuals have responsibility for structural injustice as they contribute to processes that produce unjust outcomes. By structural injustice she means that at least some of the conditions of action are not morally acceptable. We contribute by not explicitly reflecting on what we do, by not paying attention to the broad consequences of our actions, because we are busy focusing on immediate goals and outcomes. In this model of responsibility, change and reform involve many people. It is shared responsibility: a person is responsible in a partial way, and it is ultimately political responsibility.

To illustrate her model, Young effectively uses the apparel industry and the anti-sweatshop movement. She shows, for instance, how our purchasing choices (deciding what clothes we buy) contribute to supporting or diminishing sweatshops in developing nations. It can be as small a matter as that, similar to the decision to buy only fair-trade coffee. Young recognises that it may be asking too much to expect each of us to work actively to recognise and restructure each and every one of the structural injustices for which we arguably share responsibility. In looking at how we should choose the best ways to use our limited time, resources and creative energy to respond to injustice, Young claims responsibility is different from duty. There is not a specific rule of action, but more openness as to what constitutes carrying out one's responsibility. Moral agents must decide what they can and should do under the circumstances, and how to order moral priorities. We consider where our action can be most useful, or which injustices we regard as most urgent. As moral agents we each have different opportunities and capacities.

Young offers four key areas when considering these choices.

- *Interest: Where does your interest lie?* Victims of injustice, with the greatest interest in its elimination and often unique insights into social sources and probable effects of proposed change, have a responsibility, too. They are unlikely to succeed, however, without the help and support of others who are less vulnerable.
- *Power: What is your potential to act on or influence the processes that produce the outcomes of interest?* This can be soft power, such as having a voice or some influence on others. The idea is to focus where one has greater capacity to influence structural processes.
- *Privilege: Are you being privileged by some form of structural injustice?* Those who

benefit have special moral responsibilities to contribute to organised efforts to correct them, and they can adapt to changed circumstances without suffering serious deprivation.

☐ *Collective ability:* Are you connected to others through shared interests, shared power or group membership that would enable you to act collectively? There may be more influence to be had for one issue of injustice versus another.

ACTING ETHICALLY AS A NURSE IN THE GLOBAL COMMUNITY

I find this social connection model particularly helpful in my attempts to make choices related to action on global health disparities. It also explicitly places my own efforts with that of others. Nurses are the professional group most trusted by the public (Quan 2007), and we can act on this trust by influencing action on health for all. Nurse educators and researchers have the power (and the responsibility) to shape how this and the next generation of nurses understands and responds to global health problems.

Concrete ideas for action on what to do as an ethical nurse in a global community are increasingly being shared. In 2006, *Advances in Nursing Science* (ANS) put before the nursing community some ideas on global praxis and responsibility. In this issue, for instance, Adeline Falk-Rafael (2006) from York University in Canada wrote of voice, beginning her article with the motto of the LIVE 8 concert: 'We don't want your money; we want your voice.' Her point is well taken. Citizens' voices can pressure governments to meet their global commitments by increasing aid, by creating fair trade and money-lending practices; citizens can insist that their nation responds swiftly to stop genocide. Elie Wiesel (1986, p. 3) has said, 'Let us remember: what hurts the victim most is not the cruelty of the oppressor but the silence of the bystander.' We need to ask: 'How do we align our government with our hearts?' (Kristof 2006, p. 12).

Nancy Crigger and Lygia Holcomb (2007) outlined ways to promote global nursing citizenship: education that creates sensitive, reflexive nurses who are aware of their own values and culturally shaped perspectives, and of the need to attend respectfully to those of others. Nurses need education that pays attention to social justice, responsibility and global ethics in approaches to practice and research, and to be reminded that this has been a part of nursing since Nightingale's time. Verena Tschudin and Christine Schmitz (2003) had earlier pointed out that 'nurses' responsibility to prevent illness and alleviate suffering includes the morbidity caused by war'. Nurses need to be able to be active in conflict resolution and to have an understanding of their capacity to be agents of change. This has to be part of both undergraduate and continuing education.

The ICN states on its website (ICN) that it enables the 13 million nurses in the world to act collectively on global health issues. ICN is providing leadership in such ways as calling for an effectively funded UN agency for women; is working to give knowledge and training for health workers of refugee populations in Africa (among the world's most vulnerable people); fighting against counterfeit medicine; and developing strategies to deal with the global nursing shortage. It has established a nurse politician network for elected and appointed nurse politicians to communicate. As nurses, we come to our practice with an explicit responsibility to act to meet the health needs of the public, which is a responsibility unrestricted by considerations of age, colour, creed, culture, disability or illness, gender, nationality, politics, race or social status. We are grounded in a good space for addressing our responsibilities in a global community.

Although it is easy to get discouraged and overwhelmed by the senseless and needless suffering in the world, we can make a difference. The ethical demand is inherently terrifying in its call. Being anxious about it is intrinsic to being ethical. Lewis (2005) says that his work in Africa leaves him both full of rage and full of hope. This may be how it has to be for all of us for a time. This is what I will tell that young practitioner, struggling like me with both his local and global responsibilities, should the opportunity come again. I will tell him to hold to the words with which Chief Dan George (1975, p. 20) closed his letter:

> I know in your heart, you wish you could help. I wonder if there is much you can do, and yet there is a lot you can do. When you meet my children, respect each one for what he is, a child and your brother. Maybe it all boils down to that.

REFERENCES

Austin W. Nursing Ethics in an Era of Globalization. *Advances in Nursing Sciences.* 2001; **24**(2): 1–18.

Austin W. Global Health Challenges, Human Rights and Nursing Ethics. In: Storch J, Rodney P, Starzomski R, editors. *Toward a Moral Horizon: nursing ethics for leadership and practice.* Toronto: Pearson Education Canada; 2004. pp. 339–56.

Badhwar N. International Aid: when giving becomes a vice. *Social Philosophy & Policy Foundation.* 2006; **23**: 69–101.

Bauman Z. *Postmodern Ethics.* Cambridge: Basil Blackwell; 1993.

Bauman Z. *Globalization: the human consequences.* New York: Columbia University Press; 1998.

Benatar SR, Daar AS, Singer PA. Global Health Challenges: the need for an expanded discourse on bioethics. *PLoS Medicine.* 2005; **2**(7): 587–9.

Camus A. *The Plague.* New York: Vintage Books; 1947.

Camus A. *The Fall* and *Exile and the Kingdom.* O'Brien J, translator. New York: The Modern Library; 1957.

Crigger N, Holcomb L. Practical Strategies for Providing Culturally Sensitive, Ethical Care in Developing Nations. *Journal of Transcultural Nursing.* 2007; **18**(1): 70–6.

Dallaire R. *Shake Hands With the Devil: the failure of humanity in Rwanda*. Toronto: Random House Canada; 2003.

Falk-Rafael A. Globalization and Global Health: toward nursing praxis in the global community. *Advances in Nursing Science*. 2006; **29**(1): 2–14.

Freidman T. *The Lexus and the Olive Tree: understanding globalization*. New York: Farrar, Straus & Giroux; 1999.

Gaita R. *A Common Humanity: thinking about love and truth and justice*. London: Routledge; 2000.

George, Chief D. I was Born 1000 years ago . . . UNESCO Courier. 1975; **XXVIII**(1): 16–20.

Goodin R. *Protecting the Vulnerable: a reanalysis of our social responsibilities*. Chicago: University of Chicago Press; 1985.

ICN. *Code of Ethics for Nurses*. Geneva: ICN; 2006.

ICN. Available at: http://www.icn.ch/index.html (accessed 13 June 2007).

Ignatieff M. *The Warrior's Honour: ethnic war and the modern conscience*. Toronto: Penguin; 1997.

Jowitt K. *The New World Disorder*. Berkeley, CA: University of California Press; 1992.

Kristof N. The Silence of Bystanders. *The New York Times*. 19 March 2006.

Levinas E. *Collected Philosophical Papers*. Lingis A, translator. Dordrecht: Martinus Nijhoff; 1987.

Lewis S. *Race Against Time*. Toronto: House of Anansi Press; 2005.

Lovelock J. *Gaia: a new look at life on earth*. Oxford: Oxford University Press; 1979.

McLuhan M. *Understanding Media*. New York: Mentor; 1964.

Nagel T. *The View from Nowhere*. Oxford: Oxford University Press; 1986.

Nathaniel A. Moral Distress Among Nurses. American Nurses Association Center for Ethics and Human Rights. *Updates*, Spring 2002; 4.

O'Neill O. Life-boat Earth. In: Beitz CR, Cohen M, Scanlon T, Simmons AJ, editors. *A Philosophy and Public Affairs Reader*. Princeton, NJ: Princeton University Press; 1985. p. 262–81.

Pogge T. *World Poverty and Human Rights: cosmopolitan responsibilities and reforms*. Cambridge: Polity Press; 2002.

Pogge T. Real World Justice. *Journal of Ethics*. 2005; **9**(1–2): 29–53.

Quan K. Nurses are Most Honest and Ethical: Gallup poll results are in and nurses top the list again. 1 February 2007. Available at http://public-healthcare-issues.suite101.com/article.cfm/nurses_are_most_honest_and_ethical (accessed 9 June 2007).

Rawls J. *A Theory of Justice*. London: Oxford University Press; 1973.

Rawls J. *The Law of Peoples*; with *The Idea of Public Reason Revisited*. Cambridge, MA: Harvard University Press; 1999.

Ricoeur P. *Oneself as Another*. 2nd ed. Blamey K, translator. Chicago, IL: University of Chicago Press; 1992.

Rorty R. Moral Universalism and Economic Triage. *Proceedings of the Who are we? The Second UNESCO Philosophy Forum*; Paris, France. Diogenes 1996; **173**(44): 5–15.

Rorty R. *Philosophy and Social Hope*. London: Penguin Books; 1999.

Sachs J. *The End of Poverty*. New York: The Penguin Press; 2005.

Sanchez AO. Concerns and Hopes on the Threshold of the New Millennium. *Proceedings of the Forum 2000*; 1997 Sept 4; Prague, Czechoslovakia. Available at: http://www.forum2000.cz/en/projects/forum-2000-conferences/1997/transcripts1/morning-session--sept--4/ (accessed 9 June 2007).

Schopenhauer A. *On the Basis of Morality.* New York: Bobbs-Merill; 1965.

Schweitzer A. *The Philosophy of Civilization II: civilization and ethics.* 2nd ed. Campion CT, Russell CEB, translators. London: Adam & Charles Black; 1946.

Singer P. Famine, Affluence, and Morality. *Philosophy and Public Affairs.* 1972; **1**(1): 229–43 [revised edition]. Available at: http://www.utilitarian.net/singer/by/1972----.htm (accessed 9 June 2007).

The Holy Bible. King James version. Grand Rapids (MI): Zondervan Publishing House; 1995. Luke 10: 25–37.

Tschudin V, Schmitz C. The Impact of Conflict and War on International Nursing and Ethics. *Nursing Ethics.* 2003; **10**(4): 354–67.

Unger P. *Living High and Letting Die: our illusion of innocence.* New York: Oxford University Press; 1996.

Walker M. *Moral Understandings: feminist study in ethics.* New York: Routledge; 1998.

WHO. *Cumulative number of confirmed human cases of avian influenza A (H5N1) reported to WHO.* Available at: http://www.who.int/csr/disease/avian_influenza/country/cases_table_2007_06_12/en/index.html (accessed 12 June 2007).

Wiesel E. Introduction. In: Rittner C, Myers S, editors. *The Courage to Care: rescuers of Jews during the Holocaust.* New York: New York University Press, 1986.

Young I. Responsibility and Global Justice: a social connection model. *Social Philosophy and Policy.* 2006; **23**: 102–30.

Yutang L, editor and translator. *The Wisdom of Confucius.* 2nd ed. New York: Random House; 1943.

4

A global basis for nursing ethics in a culturally complex world

Richard Rowson

INTRODUCTION

There is increasing uncertainty about the ethical basis on which nurses and their organisations* should operate. The growing globalisation of nursing, nurses moving from culture to culture, and nursing organisations dealing with nurses and patients from many different societies, have all contributed to this quandary. A professional organisation cannot work effectively if its members adhere to different values; but on what values should nursing organisations base their practices? Should they, for example, simply accept the values of whatever culture is dominant in the society in which they operate, or should they strive to find values that are not specific or exclusive to any one culture? How far should managers and employers try to accommodate the culturally specific values and attitudes of nurses? This chapter is concerned with these questions.

WHAT ARE THE APPROPRIATE VALUES FOR NURSING ORGANISATIONS IN OUR CULTURALLY COMPLEX WORLD?

To answer this question, I suggest that a basic overall objective of nursing needs to be agreed on, as the appropriate values will be those that facilitate its achievement. I take a working definition of the objective of nursing to be:

> to promote the health of, and to care for, all people, regardless of their cultural affiliation, race, sexual orientation, level of disability, and so on.

---

* The term 'nursing organisations' is used in this chapter to cover all levels of nursing management in institutions and healthcare systems; also professional and labour associations for nurses.

I hope this is broadly acceptable to members of the profession, whatever their cultural affiliation. Those who do not accept it may find they disagree with ideas in this chapter.

If this objective is accepted, the crucial question is: What fundamental values facilitate this objective? Before answering this question, it is useful to identify the sort of values that would put the objective at risk. My experience in working on healthcare ethics policies in culturally complex situations indicates that it would be put at risk by values that are based on specific religious or secular perspectives. To see why this is so, consider how people come to hold their ethical views.

Broadly speaking, individuals come to their ethical views as a result of their cultural beliefs and experiences. For example, many people brought up in a religious tradition consider that God tells them – either through sacred texts, direct revelation or their religious leaders – how they ought to behave. However, people who do not believe in the same God have no reason to accept the same basis for ethics, and those who do not believe in any God have no reason to accept any God-based ethical views. For example, individuals who are convinced of the truth of the Marxist analysis of socio-economic forces see that analysis as a basis for how people should behave, whereas those who regard the analysis as flawed, reject it as an ethical foundation. In contrast, people from a secular liberal tradition think it is self-evident that human happiness is the most valuable objective to aim for, and therefore consider that we should do whatever we can to increase this happiness as much as possible. This view is not, however, accepted by those who think we should act in ways that their God says are right, regardless of whether doing so will make people as happy as possible.

These brief and simplified examples are sufficient to show that the reasons that are seen by members of one culture to justify particular ethical values are not seen to do so by members of all other cultures. Consequently, not everyone will accept the values of any one culture. If nursing were to base its global ethics on the values of one specific culture, e.g. one of the major religious traditions or one of the main secular left- or right-wing ideologies, or if nursing organisations in culturally complex societies were to adopt the ethical perspectives of the dominant culture, this would alienate those nurses, patients and members of the public who did not share the chosen cultural perspective.

Those who were alienated in this way would fear that nursing organisations would not regard their well-being as equally important as that of members of the chosen culture. Nurses from a different culture would lack confidence that they would be treated fairly by their profession, and patients from a different culture would lack trust in nurses. Yet such confidence and trust are vital elements in facilitating the objective of treating, caring for and comforting all who need nursing services.

This objective is also easier to achieve when nurses and nursing organisations have the goodwill of at least most people in their society. However, professions have the widespread goodwill of a population only if their values are generally thought to be in the interests of society as a whole, and not just of sectional interests. To secure such goodwill, the core values of nursing must be appropriate for all sections of society, not part of the culture of only one section.

Having considered the sort of values that are not appropriate for the global basis for nursing ethics, I turn now to those that are. To secure the confidence of people of all cultures, the nursing profession must make clear that it values *fairness*. Fairness requires nurses to:

- regard the interests and health of people as equally important, regardless of their cultural or religious affiliation, race, gender, sexual orientation, level of disability or lifestyle
- not discriminate between people on the basis of any culturally specific attitudes that nurses (or nursing organisations) may have
- treat individuals in ways that are appropriate and just for their specific needs, entitlements and deserts.

To enjoy the trust of patients and nurses, the nursing profession also needs to make clear that it values *autonomy* and *integrity*.

'Valuing autonomy' as used in this chapter means enabling individuals to make informed decisions with regard to how they should be treated, and respecting those decisions once they have been made. Since such decisions not only reflect individuals' understanding of the healthcare situation, but also their values and cultural views, nursing managers and employers should respect the cultural views of nurses as far as possible, and nurses should do the same to patients. Nurses should, for example, aim to give patients a good quality of life in the way they choose to live and respect how they wish to be treated.

To value integrity, members of the profession at all levels should strive to integrate their actions with their stated professional values, roles and objectives. This includes doing their best to do what they say they will do, and being honest with colleagues and patients, including admitting the limits of what they can do.

Finally, members of the profession must regard the *results* of their actions as ethically important. They must value the promotion of health and alleviation of suffering, and always be concerned to produce the most beneficial outcomes they can.

These values – fairness, respect for autonomy, integrity, and concern to achieve the best results – not only help the profession to enjoy the goodwill, trust and confidence it needs, they also give nurses an added incentive to achieve the overall objective of nursing. When nurses genuinely value being fair, they feel it is important to treat everyone well and not give less care to those for whom they have less empathy. When they value autonomy, they want to help patients to be as independent and self-determining as possible and when they think it important to bring about the best results, they have a constant incentive to do so. Finally, valuing their own integrity can help them maintain the professional standards they are credited as having.

These four values are not culturally specific, in the sense that they are not exclusive to any one religious or secular ideology. In fact, at least two of them, and in some cases all of them, are found in all the major religious and secular traditions. Consequently, they are compatible with the personal values of most people. They will also be compatible with the views of people who endorse the objective of nursing put forward at the beginning of this chapter. Indeed, some may see these values as implicit in that objective.

A FRAMEWORK OF VALUES

The four values outlined previously provide a global basis for nursing ethics that can be summarised as four principles:
- ❐ to treat people *fairly*
- ❐ to respect people's *autonomy*
- ❐ to act with *integrity*
- ❐ to seek the most beneficial *results*.

This gives the simple mnemonic: **FAIR** – Fairly, Autonomy, Integrity and Results – an easily remembered framework within which nursing decisions can be made.

This framework does not dictate what these decisions should be. Usually some consideration must be given to how the principles should be applied to particular circumstances, and sometimes the principles may clash so that decisions have to be made as to how they should be prioritised. For instance, sometimes the most beneficial results in terms of the well-being of patients can be promoted only by acting against their wishes. Sometimes the full delivery of nursing services can be maintained only by requiring nurses to take part in procedures that they would prefer to avoid, examples of which are considered below. In such cases, members of the profession, whether nurses making decisions about the treatment of patients, or managers deciding on the requirements they make of nurses, have to decide to which principle to give priority. Balancing the relative importance of such principles in particular circumstances is part of nurses' professional responsibility. As professional practitioners, they have individual discretion and may be held accountable for how they take these principles into account.

While the framework does not rob nurses and managers of their professional autonomy, it does indicate the limit and range of ethical considerations it is professionally appropriate for them to take into account. It makes clear that the values and attitudes of their personal cultural perspectives should not be part of the ethical criteria on which their decisions are based. If they were to make such decisions on the basis of their own cultural values, the confidence their patients and colleagues had in them would be betrayed. Patients should be able to trust that any nurse will give them the care and attention they need even if the nurse has a different cultural affiliation, supports a rival political party or disapproves of their lifestyle. Similarly, nurses should be able to rely on their managers and employers to treat them in accordance with values that are known and accepted throughout the profession, and not in accordance with particular cultural or sectional interests.

Although values should not be part of the criteria on which decisions in nursing are based, awareness of how nurses' actions might affect people with particular cultural views should be part of the data that is taken into account when making a decision. For example, nurses should not decide how to treat a patient on the basis of their own religious perspectives, but should take into account how a patient who has particular religious beliefs might be affected by certain practices or aspects of treatment. Similarly, a healthcare policy committee should not decide what treatments are to be made available and withdrawn on the basis of the particular religious perspectives of its members, but should consider how its proposed policies might affect members of the public who have particular religious affiliations.

TO WHAT EXTENT CAN THE NURSING PROFESSION ACCOMMODATE THE CULTURALLY SPECIFIC VIEWS OF NURSES?

In culturally complex societies the appropriateness of nurses respecting the cultural views of patients is generally accepted. However, there is less agreement as to how far nursing organisations can and should accommodate the cultural perspectives of nurses.

One cause of disagreement over this issue is the tendency of nursing organisations to make open-ended and vague commitments as employers to 'respect diversity'. This gives rise to unrealistic expectations as to how far this is possible. The rest of this chapter considers this matter by looking at various situations.

Situation 1

A Muslim nurse working in a hospital in a country where Muslims are in a minority asks permission to wear a niqab, a veil over her face. The hospital allows her to do so for a trial period to see how it affects her work. The result is that many patients, especially elderly and confused people, and children, are frightened by her because they cannot see her face. The evidence indicates that the niqab interferes with giving care and comfort to patients. The view is taken that in this case acceding to the nurse's request is less important than achieving the main objective of treating, caring for and comforting all the patients. Two of the values in the framework have been weighed against each other – respecting autonomy and seeking the best results – and one is given priority.

Had the nurse been working in a hospital in a country where people were used to the niqab, wearing it may not have interfered with bringing comfort to patients, and so the request might have been accepted. This does not, however, mean that the acceptability of a culturally specific demand is determined by whether it is a demand of the dominant culture in that society. The crucial ethical consideration is whether the request interferes with the primary objective of nursing. In a country where Muslims are in a minority, wearing the niqab was found to impede nursing care, but in a country where they are in a majority it might be different. Whether a particular request interferes with the objective of nursing sufficiently to outweigh the value of respecting a nurse's wishes may vary according to the cultural make-up of the society in which the request is made.

Situations 2 and 3

Compare the previous situation with the following ones.
1   A nurse asks permission to wear a hijab, which covers only her hair.
2   A nurse in a predominantly Muslim country asks to wear as jewellery a Star of David, a crucifix, or other religious symbol.

As in the case of the niqab, the ethical framework highlights the need to weigh the value of acceding to the nurses' requests against the likely consequences of doing so. Although in neither case would the symbols prevent the nurse relating to patients as much as the niqab might do, the question arises as to whether patients, who do not share the same cultural affiliations as the symbols represent, might fear that the nurses would be less empathic to patients who do share the affiliations.

A decision in such cases should not be made on the basis of whether the professionals who make it are sympathetic to one cultural affiliation or another. The ethical criteria on which the decision should be based, i.e. balancing the value of acceding to the request against the likely consequences of doing so, remain the same whatever the predominant culture of the situation in which it is taken. However, the data taken into account in reaching the decisions, i.e. the likely effects on patients of wearing the symbols, might vary according to the cultural affiliations of the patients.

In the following situations, where nurses' beliefs and attitudes interfere with the overall nursing objective, the views taken by management are the result of applying the values of the framework.

Situation 4

Some nurses regard the termination of pregnancy as unacceptable on religious grounds, and so do not wish to take part either in the operations or in the associated nursing procedures. The management takes the view that if the nurses can be redeployed and are able to make a full professional contribution elsewhere in the hospital, and if nursing procedures can be carried out by others who do not object to termination, the request can be granted. If not, the nurses may be required to participate in the procedures. The management view is that in these circumstances the delivery of nursing services is more important than acceding to the nurses' requests.

Situation 5

Some nurses find it difficult to comply with the professional requirement that they treat homosexual people with the same respect as they treat others because they despise what they understand as the lifestyle of homosexuals. The management suggests these nurses take a professional development course in the hope that this will increase their understanding and improve their ability to relate to homosexual patients. In the meantime, since it is not possible to ensure that these nurses never have to deal with homosexual people, they are required to put aside their attitudes and treat all people, regardless of their sexual orientation, with the same care and concern.

Situation 6

Some nurses are reluctant to spend time administering highly intensive and expensive treatment to elderly patients on the grounds that the large amount of resources absorbed by the treatment is disproportionate to the temporary benefits it produces. They argue that their time and other healthcare resources could be used more beneficially. The view of management is that since these procedures are medical policy, the nurses should not refuse to administer them on a case-by-case basis, as to do so is unfair on the particular patients with whom they happen to be working. If the nurses wish to challenge the policy, they should do so through other channels, such as their professional body.

In all these situations, nursing organisations are seen as entitled to require nurses to put aside their cultural views if their requests cannot be made compatible with the fundamental objective of nursing, the proper delivery of services and the fundamental values of the ethical framework. The view is also taken that in such circumstances nurses have a professional obligation to put aside their personal values and cultural perspectives.

Although this obligation restricts nurses' individual autonomy, the restriction is ethically acceptable on two grounds. First, as long as the nurses were aware of the values and objective of nursing when they joined the profession and therefore made an informed decision to do so, they can be regarded as having accepted this restriction voluntarily. Second, the value of the result, namely the full delivery of the nursing services, is considered on balance to justify the restriction to their autonomy in certain circumstances.

AN ETHICAL OBLIGATION OF THE NURSING PROFESSION AND OF NURSING ORGANISATIONS

If nursing organisations, managers and professional bodies accept the global basis for nursing ethics put forward in this chapter, they should also accept that they have an obligation to make clear the core values and objectives of nursing to people who are considering joining the profession, as well as to those who may become patients.

As employers, they should also make clear that, although they will respect the cultural views of their employees as much as possible, they can do so only as long as this does not prevent them from fulfilling their essential obligations to people who need their services. In particular, they should explicitly state that they cannot give an open-ended commitment to 'respect diversity'.

CONCLUSION

In this chapter, I have put forward values for a global basis for nursing ethics that should be broadly acceptable to people from the major religious and secular traditions. These values constitute an ethical framework that is both practical, in that it gives an easily memorable checklist of ethical concerns to be taken into account when decisions are made, and respectful, in that it gives professionals the scope to reach their own judgements on how to relate the values to specific conditions.

If these values were adopted as the global ethical basis for nursing, nursing organisations and nurses in all cultures and societies would have an agreed-on and acknowledged framework within which to debate ethical issues. Having such a framework would be supportive in many ways.

❑ It would enable professionals to identify quickly those aspects of a situation that are ethically significant.

❑ It would give colleagues a shorthand way of referring to these aspects, and a common conceptual structure within which to discuss them.

❑ When people were uncertain what they ought to do, it would help them to identify the reasons for their uncertainty – such as the clashing of two principles – and pinpoint the issues they need to think through to reach a decision.

❑ It would provide an ethical remit for people to focus on, thereby helping to ensure that they do not make evaluative judgements from the point of view of particular religious or secular bases.

❑ It would remind people of considerations they may have overlooked and that others may expect them to take into account.

Questions to consider

Are the four values of the framework compatible with your own religious or secular cultural perspectives?

If they are not, over what points do they diverge?

What difficulties do you see in adopting the suggested values as the global ethical basis for nursing?

Do you think it would be possible to overcome these difficulties?

5

Values at the heart of addiction in a globalised world

Mary Tod Gray

INTRODUCTION

Drug addiction* is a global phenomenon, which both reveals and threatens the experience of freedom and power. Freedom and power are values that assume dominance in the growing pandemic of addictions as the forces of globalisation change the expectations of individuals and societies, and their relationships to one another. In this chapter, I explore how these values can be discerned within the subjective experiences of the individual addicted to drugs, the dynamics of the nurse–client relationship, and the social context of the global drug trade. Such discernment elicits new directions for nursing approaches to the human qualities in addiction.

Freedom and power examined in the context of drug addiction reveal human values that transcend national boundaries. These values impart meaning to the clients' and nurses' responses to the dynamics of the nurse–client relationship. They give direction to therapeutic and sustainable client goals. On a global scale, nurses seek realistic solutions to the suffering experienced in addiction by clients and societies. These realistic solutions emerge from a values perspective attuned to the experience of freedom and power at the heart of addiction.

FREEDOM AND POWER: THE INDIVIDUAL ABUSING DRUGS

Freedom is a concept that originates from a feeling. That feeling is one of unfettered motion that the individual experiences internally. This motion both links the individual to and liberates the individual from his or her world.† The individual perceives this feeling of movement by its change in intensity and

---

* Addiction and substance abuse are used interchangeably in this chapter. Drugs refer to illegal psychotropic drugs; the most common are heroin, cocaine, methamphetamines and marijuana.

† See Mary Tod Gray (2007) for a more in-depth discussion.

interruption of ongoing sensations.* The more tightly constricted the previous sense of movement, the more sharply the individual contrasts and values a sense of liberated motion. Children racing from the confines of the classroom at the end of the school day visually exemplify this contrast in perceived feelings of motion. In this light, the individual assigns the feeling of movement a positive or negative value, according to its contrast with preceding feelings.

Movement impeded by obstacles, boundaries, rules, or constraints, translates to feelings of tension, resistance and limits on freedom. Feelings of power arise from actions chosen to overcome these limits. Choice in this instance denotes the ability to direct movement towards a goal directly tied to survival or indirectly to a goal highly valued by the individual. Feelings of power derived from choice developmentally connect to individuation and autonomy. From this developmental bedrock, feelings of power energise the actualisation of individual potential, and tightly connect to feeling free to move towards a chosen goal. Individuals value freedom and power as expressions of their uniqueness.†

Narratives from individuals abusing psychoactive substances (Gray 2004, 2005, 2007) express both the feelings of unfettered freedom and of power resulting from choice: movement forward towards a goal, or to overcome obstacles to that goal. Drug narratives cite feelings of freedom and power as they connect to an intensified sense of individuality. In contrast, but equally salient, some drug narratives express a burden of self and individuality followed by a heightened sense of connection to others or a universal source such as God, energy, or a transcendent being (Gray 2003, 2004, 2005). Psychoactive substances then become important as they prompt the experience of, or diminish obstacles to, these valued universal feelings: in some ways to feel unique and powerful, and in some ways connected and safe. The individual chooses.

FREEDOM AND POWER: THE NURSE–CLIENT RELATIONSHIP

Freedom and power in the context of individual drug experience influence the nurse–client relationship in two ways. First, the client relinquishes the feelings of freedom and power experienced with drugs when he or she enters or is forced into treatment and a drug-free environment. The client relinquishes a part of the

---

* William James (1890/1981) described the perception of body changes as they occur as emotions, characterised as 'seizures of excitement'. More recently, Michael Lyvers (2000) and George Lowenstein (1999) have detailed the links between physiological changes and emotions in drug addictions.

† Susan Leddy (2006) notes that, in Eastern cultures, choice is indirect and power derives from family and community belonging rather than individuation. The amalgamating effects of globalisation have already begun to change this relationship between individual and cultural traditions in East Asian countries (Friedman 2005).

power of self found in isolation and individuation when he or she accepts the feeling of connection encountered in the professional response and responsibility to the client. The bond of trust, which represents this feeling of connection, forms the foundation on which new experiences of self and a sense of safety can be created, and in which freedom and power can be experienced in drug-free life-styles.

Second, and often unrecognised, the nurse, too, must struggle with issues of freedom and power in the relationship's context and its long-term outcomes. While the client experiences freedom and power primarily during drug experiences and not in sobriety, the nurse experiences freedom and power through the dynamics of the relationship. The nurse's professional power rests on assumptions of responsibility when the drug-abusing client presents with changes in mental status, physical debility, lack of insight, or poor choices that threaten health. The nurse directs changes in behaviour towards health outcomes and social norms. This direction is often experienced by the client addicted to drugs as control: a sensible threat to freedom and personal power induced by intimations of feeling controlled by the power of others, in this instance the nurse.

Sustainable health outcomes occur when both the client and the nurse consider the risks to the sense of freedom and choice that the therapeutic relationship and programme entail. The feelings at the heart of freedom and power have often been elusive in sobriety for the individual addicted to drugs. The client relinquishes those feelings, when first giving up drugs, and potentially when entering into the feelings of connection in the nurse–client relationship. The client feels restricted and impotent instead of free and powerful. For the client the long-term risk and fear is that the therapeutic programme fails to restore the feelings underpinning freedom and power. Without these feelings, which express the client's values, such a programme is difficult to sustain.

The risk for the nurse is that the client addicted to drugs is vulnerable and sensitive to threats to personal freedom and power of choice. Unless the nurse has examined these concepts in the light of the addiction process, he or she fails to build the programme of recovery on values fundamental to the addiction problem. The nurse equally risks projecting a sense of moral superiority that follows from the professional norms and mores that the nurse represents. The client struggles with perceived threats to freedom and power, evident in his or her resistance to social norms or conventional solutions to the drug problem. Part of the client's sense of power might even reside in this resistance to social norms as a source of empowerment.

For the nurse to help the client build solutions that embrace sustainable experiences of freedom and power, he or she must recognise and relinquish power resting in received authority or a sense of moral superiority. To do this requires that the nurse who works with addicted clients must be acutely sensitive to his or her own sense of freedom and power derived from the professional relationship. Too often, the nurse, denied professional autonomy in healthcare system decisions has little experience with professional power except in the context of the client relationship. He or she might therefore have little insight into the client's response to his or her projected power in that relationship.* Relinquishing power to the client frees the nurse from standardised social responses that neglect the affective values at the core of addiction.

FREEDOM AND POWER IN THE CONTEXT OF THE GLOBAL DRUG TRADE

If freedom and power colour the perceptions of the relationship between the client and nurse, they pervade the context of addiction: the global drug trade. Drugs are valued commodities in the global market as drug sales provide access to resources of freedom and power. Economically, freedom involves investment and participation in the fruits of one's work; power represents choice in relation to distribution of society's resources. From this perspective, the illegal drug trade symbolises an instrument by which these values can materialise and prosperity can be extended. In the global market, drug sales are likely to represent a living income.

From a political perspective, the drug trade represents a means to wrest power from dominant groups and seize it for local or minority groups. In Asia, revolutionaries seeking to overthrow tyranny and gain political power use the profits from the illegal drug trade to purchase arms towards this end (Thai Press Report 2005). In Afghanistan, the sale of illegal drugs is tied to financing terrorists who threaten the stability of governments and hegemony of world powers (Chalk 2000; Mann *et al.* 2006). On the streets of New York (Fullilove *et al.* 1998) or Dublin (Lally 2005), disenfranchised teenage gangs unite and claim territories financed by illegal drug sales. The lucrative drug trade entices indigenous populations struggling for subsistence to farm marijuana (Clayton 1995), poppies (Wodak *et al.* 2004) or coca plants (Guarcy 2001; Huggler 2005).

Paradoxically, the fruits of globalisation that offer interconnectivity between populations in the world have also opened new paths to the illegal drug trade and an increase in global drug traffic. Efficient transportation and communication technology, such as the Internet and cell phone, rapidly connect drug buyers

---

* Clients with addiction problems are often described by healthcare professionals as 'manipulative'. This conveys two perspectives: one, the client is taking action (however ineffectual) to redress a lost sense of power in the relationship; and two, the nurse is responding to the perceived threat to his or her power by describing the client's behaviour in terms that both distance the professional and belittle the client.

and sellers across the world undetected. The military and police, directed by national and international policies, combat this drug trade with mixed results. Intravenous drug use has increased and facilitated pandemics of blood-borne diseases such as AIDS and hepatitis, straining already insufficient public health resources. Interconnectivity has also fostered widespread awareness of disparity in incomes, and decreased opportunities for employment and education (Wodak & Crofts 1993; Wodak *et al.* 2004). The latter engenders a widespread sense of freedom denied and choices constrained.

Globally, illegal drug production and sales exploit the hopes of the poor and disenfranchised people for freedom and empowerment; the drug market capitalises on their vulnerabilities. Minority groups, illegal immigrants, subsistence farmers and prostitutes use and are used by the drug trade as they seek access to a better life on Native American reservations (Kershaw 2006), in Appalachia (Clayton 1995), Nigeria and Brazil (Guarcy 2001), Bolivia (Forero 2006), or Asia's Golden Triangle and Golden Crescent (Chalk 2000). Drug lords in international cartels use the drug trade's enormous profits to purchase guns, launder money, corrupt government officials and agencies, and ultimately perpetuate terror and terrorism (Chalk 2000; Naím 2005). Bartering sex for drugs (Ellwood & Williams 1997; Green *et al.* 2005) transmits disease and human degradation. It also symbolises the paradox of addiction: enslavement to the very commodity through which freedom and power are pursued.

IMPLICATIONS FOR NURSING IN THE GLOBAL CONTEXT OF ADDICTION

Nursing practice at its best recognises the 'free spirit' in human suffering; it operates from a premise that drug addiction is not a passive state visited upon a victim, but a metaphor for the multiple layers of meaning that emerge as drug addiction interacts with globalisation.* One of the special skills that nurses offer to individuals addicted to drugs is to help them uncover the meaning that illness creates in life.† Exploring experiences of freedom and choice provide both an ethical and conceptual framework for a nursing practice that accentuates the affective values in illness and offers choice as a basis for healing in addiction (Chopra 1997), a guide to healthiness (Leddy 2006) and a deterrent to the numbing forces of consumerism (Barber 2001; Walton 2001).

Global consumerism introduces a uniformity that threatens the rich diversity

---

* Susan Sontag discussed illness as a metaphor in relation to tuberculosis and cancer (1978), and AIDS (1989).

† The meaning that illness creates in life has been explored in literature, social commentary and nursing (Mann 1953; Sontag 1978, 1989; Newman 1994).

found in the traditions, beliefs and rituals of the many world cultures (Barber 2001). Modern addictions in general coincide with a loss of the community rituals and traditions that give meaning to our lives (Wilshire 1998). Nurses can counter these losses and sense of anomie arising from uniformity because they work at the local level with individuals and communities. They devise health strategies that respect and incorporate personal and cultural values at the heart of liberating and empowered feelings. These ideas are not new. What is new is the insertion of these ideas into the political process and policies that direct the response to public health issues such as addiction.

Awareness of the wonderful opportunities that globalisation affords must be equally tempered with the threats to public health that its opportunities create.* Advances in technology and access to diverse commodities offered in the global market provide endless choices; the freedom afforded by endless choice for its own sake is meaningless without an acknowledged goal, from which the individual and community draw purpose and a meaning that unite them in a common good. Nurses working with communities on standards of living will lessen the pull of growing poppies in Afghanistan, growing coca in Columbia and Bolivia, or growing marijuana in Kentucky. Nurses who educate individuals, local communities, and their leaders with the tools for peaceful change at the local level provide practice for their participation in larger changes in national and international governing structures. Nurses who join the public policy table speak from a public health perspective. Such a perspective invites a more realistic and ultimately sustainable approach to addicted individuals and the social costs of addiction;† it recognises and addresses the underlying economic and political inequities that fuel the illegal drug trade.

Human desires for freedom and power are fertile grounds for the best and worst actions of individuals and societies. In a globalised world, nurses can no longer limit their focus to the client and the nurse–client relationship. Health issues such as addiction must be examined, and strategies devised within a global context. Several thoughts are offered to spur this global perspective.

---

* Threats to public health include violence connected to the drug trade, sex for drugs and resulting sexually transmitted diseases, intravenous drugs and resulting blood-borne diseases: AIDS, hepatitis, and risks to immigrants who transport illegal drugs in body cavities.

† Ann Roche and Keith Evans's (2000) integrated intervention drug model proposes a national (Australia) drug policy that offers a variety of health-directed choices: harm reduction, use reduction, non-use and abstinence. Such choices capitalise on the individual's capacity for change through a variety of paths. Another creative option emerges in Rotterdam's efforts to regulate the hard drug trade (Van De Mheen & Gruter 2004). Here, both government and private organisations have collaborated to introduce 'reporting centers for drug-related nuisance . . . and "self-regulation" of dealing addresses and drug consumption/selling rooms' among others (p. 1). Such public policy acknowledges the drug trade's organisation and capacity to self-regulate.

1   Drugs, while a tangible, material good, are also an idea-based good (Friedman 2005). As a commodity, drugs are valued by both health professionals and the public. Whoever controls a valued good acquires feelings of freedom and power. Those who control drug prescriptions, administration, and trade benefit from the power of drugs as an idea of health, healing and relief from suffering. Respect and status accord to those who provide, prescribe or administer drugs within a community. This includes not just health professionals but drug dealers, drug lords, shaman, and traditional healers, as well as addicted individuals who self-medicate (Khantzian 1985).

2   Power arises not only from the money generated in the legal and illegal sale of drugs, but also from the political influence that the money buys indirectly or directly in government policies. In many countries, money from the drug trade provides social welfare for the poor when its government cannot, obscuring the moral divide between good and bad (Naím 2005). Nurses, who recognise the privation and deprivation that spur individuals or indigenous people's involvement with the drug trade, must raise community awareness of the risks for manipulation, degradation and oppression arising from drug trade involvement. More proactively, they must tackle the tougher problems of fostering an infrastructure that provides meaningful work to give a sense of freedom and power to people's lives.

3   The global community of nursing professionals cannot limit themselves to advocacy for the vulnerable; they must become provocateurs, arousing feelings of movement described as freedom, and action envisioned as power that pervade the phenomenon of addiction as described above. They are not just speaking for the vulnerable, but stimulating changes in the broader system. A provocateur's courage entails risk, because stimulating feelings of action cannot guarantee that outcomes will be orderly and prescribed, or that political processes can be harnessed behind the right horse.

4   The illegal drug trade is inextricable from the social crises accentuated by globalisation. Nurses must be able to see a phenomenon such as addiction for the human values its affliction represents and the global context that simultaneously reveals and supports its presence. The question then becomes: How does the global nursing community develop its skills as provocateurs, to move others toward a global justice that honours both the feelings of freedom and the power of choice as values discerned in the heart of addiction?

REFERENCES

Barber BR. *Jihad vs McWorld: terrorism's challenge to democracy*. New York: Ballantine Books; 2001.

Chalk P. The Global Heroin and Cocaine Trade. In: Stokes G, Chalk P, Gillen K. *Drugs and Democracy: in search of new directions*. Victoria, Australia: Melbourne University Press; 2000. pp. 15–35.

Chopra D. *Overcoming Addictions: the spiritual solutions*. New York: Harmony Books; 1997.

Clayton RR. *Marijuana in the 'Third World': Appalachia, USA*. Boulder, CO: Lynne Rienner Publishers; 1995.

Ellwood WN, Williams ML. Powerlessness and HIV Prevention Among People Who Trade Sex for Drugs ('Strawberries'). *AIDS Care*. 1997; **9**(3): 273–85. Available at: http://web22.epnet.com/DeliveryPrintSave.asp? (accessed 10 February 2006).

Forero J. Bolivia's Knot: no to cocaine, but yes to coca. *The New York Times*. 2006. Available at: http://www.nytimes.com/2006/02/12/international/americas/12Bolivia.html? (accessed 12 February 2006).

Friedman TL. *The World is Flat*. New York: Farrar, Straus & Giroux; 2005.

Fullilove MT, Heron V, Jimenez W, *et al*. Injury and Anomie: effects of violence on an inner-city community. *American Journal of Public Health*. 1998; **88**(6): 924–7. Available at: http://web.ebscohost.com/ehost/pdf?vid=3&hid=6&sid=5e4ccca4-8f8b-416f-a126-288ad88d00ab%40SRCSM2 (accessed 18 April 2008).

Gray MT. Feelings of Relation in the Fringe of Consciousness: implications for the subjective experience of addiction and the nurse–client relationship. *Archives of Psychiatric Nursing*. 2003; **17**(5): 237–43.

Gray MT. Philosophical Inquiry: an argument for radical empiricism as a philosophical framework for the phenomenology of addiction. *Qualitative Health Research*. 2004; **14**(8): 1151–64.

Gray MT. The Shifting Sands of Self: a framework for the experience of self in addiction. *Nursing Philosophy*. 2005; **6**: 119–30.

Gray MT. Freedom and Resistance: the phenomenal will in addiction. *Nursing Philosophy*. 2007; **8**: 3–15.

Green LL, Fullilove MT, Fullilove RE. Remembering the Lizard: reconstructing sexuality in the rooms of narcotics anonymous. *Journal of Sex Research*. 2005; **42**(1): 28–34. Available at: http://web.ebscohost.com/ehost/pdf?vid=12&hid=8sid=7e4ebaac-8tbb-4c1e-b678-7ed2b453aab5%40SRCSm1 (accessed 18 April 2008).

Guarcy M. Money and the International Drug Trade in Sao Paulo. *International Social Science Journal*. 2001; **53**(169): 379–86.

Huggler J. Afghan Minister Quits Over Opium Trade. *The Independent*. 28 September 2005. Available at: http://web.lexis-nexis.com/universe/document? (accessed 27 February 2006).

James W. *The Principles of Psychology*. Vols 1–2. Cambridge, MA: Harvard University Press; 1890/1891.

Kershaw S. Dizzying Rise and Abrupt Fall for a Reservation Drug Dealer. *The New York Times*. 2006. Available at: http://www.nytimes.com/2006/02/20/national/20gena.html? (accessed 20 February 2006).

Khantzian E. The Self-medication Hypothesis of Addiction Disorders. *American Journal of Psychiatry.* 1985; **142**: 1259–64.

Khantzian E. The Self-medication Hypothesis of Substance Use Disorders: a reconsideration and recent applications. *Harvard Review of Psychiatry.* 1997; **4**: 231–44.

Lally C. Illegal Drug Trade Worth EUR 1bn Here. *The Irish Times.* 30 December 2005. Available at: http://web.lexis-nexis.com/universe/document (accessed 27 February 2006).

Leddy SK. *Health Promotion: mobilizing strengths to enhance health, wellness, and well-being.* Philadelphia: F A Davis Company; 2006.

Lowenstein G. A Visceral Account of Addiction. In: Elster J, Skog OJ, editors. *Getting Hooked: rationality and addiction.* Cambridge: Cambridge University Press; 1999. pp. 235–64.

Lyvers M. A Loss of Control in Alcoholism and Drug Addiction: a neuroscientific interpretation. *Experimental and Clinical Psychopharmacology.* 2000; **8**(2): 225–49.

Mann J, Rivers D, Cooper A. Global War on Drugs. *CNN International Insight.* 1 February 2006. Available at: http://web.lexis-nexis.com/universe/document? (accessed 27 February 2006).

Mann T. *The Magic Mountain.* [Der Zauberberg]. Lowe-Porter HT, translator. New York: Knopf; 1953.

Naím M. *Illicit: how traffickers, and copycats are hijacking the global economy.* New York: Doubleday; 2005.

Newman MA. *Health as Expanding Consciousness.* 2nd ed. New York: National League for Nursing Press; 1994.

Roche A, Evans K. Harm Reduction: Integrated intervention drug model. In: Stokes G, Chalk P, Gillen K, editors. *Drugs and Democracy: in search of new directions.* Victoria, Australia: Melbourne University Press; 2000. pp. 149–62.

Sontag S. *Illness as Metaphor.* New York: Farrar, Straus & Giroux; 1978.

Sontag S. *AIDS and its Metaphors.* New York: Farrar, Straus & Giroux; 1989.

Thai Press Report. US orders assets of 11 Thais and 16 Thai companies frozen on allegations of links to Myanmar (Burma) illegal drug trade. Global NewsWire, Asia Africa Intelligence Wire, Financial Times Information. 8 November 2005. Available at: http://web.lexis-nexix.com/universe/document? (accessed 27 February 2006).

Van De Mheen D, Gruter P. Interventions on the supply side of the local hard drug market: toward a regulated hard drug trade? The case of the city of Rotterdam. *Journal of Drug Issues.* 2004; **34**(1), 145–61.

Walton S. *Out of It: a cultural history of intoxication.* London: Hamish Hamilton; 2001.

Wilshire B. *Wild Hunger: the primal roots of addiction.* New York: Rowman & Littlefield; 1998.

Wodak A, Crofts N. HIV Infection Among Injecting Drug Users in Asia: an evolving public health crisis. *AIDS Care.* 1993; **5**(3): 313–21.

Wodak A, Sarkar S, Mesquita F. The Globalization of Drug Injecting. *Addiction.* 2004; **99**: 799–801.

6

The right to health: global challenges and opportunities for nurses

Mark Chamberlain, Dominique Le Touze, James Welsh

INTRODUCTION

Both health and the right to health are increasingly seen within a global framework. This chapter develops particular themes that have been articulated in an earlier report (Amnesty International 2006), and examines the legal obligations placed on states in realising the right to health, and the ways in which this might inform the practice of nurses who are the main providers of healthcare in most regions of the world. The chapter then focuses in detail on the rights underpinning Millennium Development Goal 6 (combating HIV/AIDS) before concluding with some recommendations that aim to enhance the role of nurses in promoting the realisation of the right to health.

The right to health is a shorthand expression for the right that has been enshrined in several international and regional treaties and at least 100 national constitutions (World Health Organization 2002a). For example, the Constitution of South Africa states that: 'Everyone has the right to have access to . . . health care services, including reproductive health care' and 'no one may be refused emergency medical treatment' (South Africa 1996).

Reference to the right to health is found in several international treaties, notably in the International Covenant on Economic, Social and Cultural Rights (ICESCR 1966), to which more than 150 countries are party.* Article 12 of this covenant states in paragraph 1 that: 'States Parties . . . recognize the right of everyone to the enjoyment of the highest attainable standard of physical and mental health.' The covenant offers some suggestions on how this simple statement should be understood. However, the Committee on Economic, Social and Cultural Rights (CESCR 2000) sets out a more detailed and authoritative

---

* Treaty ratifications are available online at: http://www.unhchr.ch/tbs/doc.nsf/Statusfrset.

interpretation of the content of Article 12.* According to this statement, the right to health 'is not to be understood as a right to be healthy', but rather should be seen as containing both freedoms and entitlements. Freedoms include the right to control one's health and body, including sexual and reproductive functions; as well as rights related to physical integrity, such as the right to be free from torture, non-consensual medical treatment and experimentation. By contrast, entitlements include the right to a health system that provides all individuals with equal opportunity to enjoy the highest attainable level of health (CESCR 2000, para. 8).

In summary:

> the right to health must be understood as a right to the enjoyment of a variety of facilities, goods, services and conditions necessary for the realization of the highest attainable standard of health (CESCR 2000, para. 9).

The right to health should be understood as extending beyond healthcare to 'the underlying determinants of health, such as access to safe and potable water and adequate sanitation, an adequate supply of safe food, nutrition and housing, healthy occupational and environmental conditions, and access to health-related education and information, including on sexual and reproductive health' (CESCR 2000, para. 11).

The right to health contains the following interrelated and essential elements:

Availability. Healthcare has to be available in sufficient quantity. This is dependent on numerous factors, including: the national income; the underlying determinants of health noted above; hospitals, clinics and other health-related buildings; trained medical and professional personnel receiving domestically competitive salaries; and availability of essential drugs, as defined by the WHO Action Programme on Essential Drugs (CESCR 2000 para. 12a).

Accessibility. Health facilities, goods and services have to be accessible to everyone without discrimination. Services should:
- ❑ have a policy of non-discrimination in law and practice
- ❑ be physically accessible (including for marginalised peoples and people with disabilities)

---

* The committee is composed of 18 independent experts appointed as individuals rather than as national representatives. Their interpretative comment, General Comment 14, on the right to health represents an authoritative statement of what the right to health encompasses. See CESCR (2000).

❐ be economically accessible (affordable), whether privately or publicly provided

❐ enable accessibility of information, including the right to seek, receive and impart information, consistent with confidentiality of personal data.

Acceptability. All health facilities, goods and services must be respectful of medical ethics and culturally appropriate.

Quality. Health facilities, goods and services should be informed by best practice medical and scientific guidelines, and be quality assured.

The specific obligations on states to realise human rights, including the right to health, are threefold:

The obligation to respect. Human rights to respect require that states refrain from interfering directly or indirectly with people's enjoyment of human rights.

The obligation to protect. States must prevent, investigate, punish and ensure redress for the harm caused by abuses of human rights by third parties, private individuals, commercial enterprises or other non-state actors.

The obligation to fulfil. States need to take legislative, administrative, budgetary, judicial and other steps towards the full realisation of human rights. Governments must give priority to meeting the minimum essential levels of each right, especially for the most vulnerable people.

While states are required to take appropriate immediate action regarding their obligations to respect and protect human rights, many of the obligations imposed by the right to health arise from the 'obligation to fulfil', which requires that states meet their obligations progressively. That is, states are obliged to assure increasing realisation of this right. CESCR commented that: 'any deliberately retrogressive measures . . . would require the most careful consideration and would need to be fully justified by reference to the totality of the rights provided for in the Covenant and in the context of the full use of the maximum available resources' (1990).

By ratifying the International Covenant on Economic, Social and Cultural Rights, states agree to periodic examination by the committee overseeing the covenant regarding progress to achieving the rights within it. This process allows non-governmental organisations (NGOs) to submit their own 'shadow reports', which are often used by the committee to inform the questions they ask.

A number of UK organisations, for example, made a joint submission on the right to health in the UK when the UK government appeared before the committee in 2002 (CESCR 2002). Organisations included Doctors for Human Rights UK (formerly Physicians for Human Rights UK), the Royal College of Nursing, and other NGOs working in the area of health and human rights. These shadow reports, apart from creating an increased awareness of economic, social and cultural rights, can result in the committee issuing specific conclusions that can later be taken up by campaigning groups, as several organisations in Northern Ireland found when they took the opportunity to submit their own shadow reports. As one writer later stated (Beirne 2005):

> Trade unions, local NGOs and wider civil society were now made aware of the existence of a covenant guaranteeing social, economic and cultural rights, of the Government's obligations in this regard and of the opportunity provided by the UN monitoring process to bring about improvements. Accordingly, the UN received a number of submissions from and about Northern Ireland, which facilitated their assessment of the Government's assertions and led them to make a series of recommendations of particular relevance to the jurisdiction.

NON-DISCRIMINATION, EQUALITY AND THE RIGHT TO HEALTH

> Whatever form . . . discrimination takes, at its heart is a failure to respect the inherent rights and dignity of the person or group in question.
>
> (Khan 2004)

The right to health must be based on a principle of non-discrimination. The CESCR (2000) has clarified that discrimination is prohibited on 'grounds of race, colour, sex, language, religion, political or other opinion, nation or social origin, property, birth, physical or mental disability, health status (including HIV/ AIDS), sexual orientation and civil, political, social or other status, which has the intention or effect of nullifying or impairing the equal enjoyment or exercise of the right to health.' It is this prohibition that underpins all other human rights. The principle of non-discrimination is also linked to that of equality, the right to enjoy human rights on an equal basis. These principles supplement the ethical standards that require health professionals to provide care without discrimination and with the well-being of the individual as the foremost requirement.

Discrimination frequently prevents individuals and groups in great need from accessing or obtaining necessary care. However, this has wider ramifications for those discriminated against, including preventing or impeding their participation in the development of health policy, their access to information and to sharing the benefits of scientific developments. Recognising the serious adverse effects of discrimination on women, including their health, the UN General Assembly adopted in 1979 the Convention on the Elimination of All Forms of Discrimination Against Women (CEDAW 1979). Articles 10, 12 and 14 of the convention relate specifically to health, and the elimination of discrimination, and the promotion of equality for women in healthcare and education.

The committee charged with overseeing the convention (the CEDAW Committee (1992)) has emphasised that 'Gender-based violence is a form of discrimination that seriously inhibits women's ability to enjoy rights and freedoms on a basis of equality with men.' Nurses should be aware of how their work environment, the health system within which they operate, and their own views can be instrumental in discrimination against patients. One report (Kim & Motsei 2002) makes reference to the way some primary healthcare nurses in South Africa perceive gender-based violence as a 'cultural norm', arguably reflecting the fact that nurses share the same social environment, and experience the same levels of violence as the patients they treat. In Turkey, researchers found that more than 80% of the nurses and midwives they surveyed said that they had been present during a hymen examination carried out to determine the subject's virginity; just over half the participants indicated that virginity was important and more than half disapproved of premarital sexual relations (Gürsoy & Vural 2003). In some countries, nurses deny unmarried adolescents information about or supplies of contraceptives, although married adolescents would receive them without question (Center for Reproductive Law and Policy 2002). Racial discrimination has also been cited as a barrier to access to care for many sectors of the population (McKenzie 2003, Smedley et al. 2003).

NURSING PERSONNEL AND THE RIGHT TO THE HIGHEST ATTAINABLE STANDARD OF HEALTH

Nurses are key actors in respecting, protecting and fulfilling the right to health, as they provide a link between the healthcare system and the patient. In carrying out their work, nurses should be able to provide healthcare and treatment that is physically and economically accessible, non-discriminatory, culturally appropriate and of a high quality. While the ICESCR places an obligation on governments to ensure that these conditions prevail (CESCR 2000), health professionals, including nurses and their associations, have commitments to ethical and effective care (ICN 2006) in addition to human rights responsibilities.

Where such services are not publicly funded, governments have a responsibility to ensure health services are accessible to all, in particular healthcare relating to the gender-specific health needs of women and disadvantaged groups (Amnesty International 2005; ICN 2001a). States are obliged under Article 12 of CEDAW to 'ensure, on a basis of equality of men and women, access to health care services, including those related to family planning.'

ICN (2000) has argued that nurses should advocate policies that give priority to the health needs of the poor and other 'at risk' groups, while supporting the development of models for local health systems that reach those most in need of healthcare.

The functioning of a private sector in healthcare does not relieve the state of its obligations to respect, protect and fulfil the right to health. CESCR (2000) has noted that payment for healthcare services 'has to be based on the principle of equity, ensuring that these services, whether privately or publicly provided, are affordable for all, including socially disadvantaged groups' (para. 12b). The committee also stresses 'the need to ensure that not only the public health sector but also private providers of health services and facilities comply with the principle of non-discrimination in relation to persons with disabilities' (para. 26). The Committee on the Rights of the Child (CRC) has affirmed the duty of the state to assure the right to health where the non-state sector plays a role in healthcare delivery. In General Comment 5, the CRC emphasises 'that States parties to the Convention have a legal obligation to respect and ensure that the rights of children as stipulated in the Convention, which includes the obligation to ensure that non-State service providers operate in accordance with its provisions, thus creating indirect obligations on such actors' (2003).

An aspect of globalisation that presents a major challenge for healthcare systems is the growing migration of skilled health personnel from low- to high-income countries (de Mesquita & Gordon 2005). At the same time, the distribution of trained nurses within states is often uneven (CEDAW 1979, article 14.2b). For example, according to a recent survey of registered nurses in Malawi, 94% worked in urban areas (Muula et al. 2003)

MILLENNIUM DEVELOPMENT GOALS (2000)

> We believe that the central challenge we face today is to ensure that globalization becomes a positive force for all the world's people. For while globalization offers great opportunities, at present its benefits are very unevenly shared, while its costs are unevenly distributed. We recognize that developing countries and countries with economies in transition face special difficulties in responding to this central challenge (UN 2000).

Arising from the Millennium Declaration, the international community agreed on the Millennium Development Goals (MDGs), most of which relate directly or indirectly to health, and these are setting the agenda for global development targets.*

With each MDG linked to specific time-limited targets and indicators, progress towards achieving these goals can be monitored and governments held to account.

NURSING AND THE MILLENNIUM DEVELOPMENT GOALS

According to WHO (2002b), the contribution of nursing to the achievement of the health-related MDGs includes:

❑ monitoring poverty, by documenting the prevalence of underweight children, child and maternal mortality
❑ promoting gender equality, by educating girls and women about health issues
❑ reducing child and maternal mortality, by delivering maternal and child health services
❑ combating HIV/AIDS, malaria and other disease, by lowering their prevalence through activities directed towards prevention and treatment and reducing stigma and discrimination.

The value for nursing of an approach to health based on human rights can be illustrated by looking at the effort to combat HIV/AIDS, part of MDG 6.

MILLENNIUM DEVELOPMENT GOAL 6

MDG 6 commits the international community to 'Combat HIV/AIDS, malaria and other diseases' and reduce the burden of disease by 2015. Lack of accurate information and stigma surrounding HIV/AIDS are present across the world, partly due to taboos associated with sexual activity between men, sex involving young people, commercial and extra-marital sex, and injecting drug use. Inadequate knowledge of the disease, counter-productive laws and lack of power in relationships lead to insufficient access to HIV prevention services and an inability, particularly on the part of women, to negotiate safer sex (UNAIDS 2005a).

The human rights dimension of HIV/AIDS was recognised very early on in the pandemic, with the WHO Global Programme on AIDS taking a lead on

---

* Millennium goals touching on health include: 1. Eradicate extreme poverty and hunger, 4. Reduce child mortality, 5. Improve maternal health, 6. Combat HIV/AIDS, malaria and other diseases. Goals 2, 3, 7 and 8 on education, gender equality, environment and a global partnership also have implications for health.

promoting the protection of the rights of people living with HIV/AIDS. UN and NGO publications have reflected a concern for human rights, and protecting basic rights is widely seen as an essential component of an effective global HIV response (Amnesty International 2004).*

Health professionals are not immune from prejudice (Surlis & Hyde 2001), and people seeking care for HIV-related problems are known to have experienced stigma and discrimination within the health sector. The PAHO (2003) has noted that, despite some reduction in HIV/AIDS-related discrimination in the region, some forms of stigma that preceded the epidemic, such as homophobia, remain strong.

At the same time, nurses and midwives face the same risk of exposure to disease as their patients. In high-prevalence areas, health personnel usually have high levels of infection. A study by the Tanzanian Registration Council (*see* Chapter 8) showed that of health workers who died while registered, 67% had AIDS; for medical attendants figures were 77%, and for nurses 53%.

Nurses and midwives in professional practice treating patients with HIV/AIDS are faced with a number of treatment challenges. All nurses can play a part in advocating for the rights of HIV/AIDS patients and combating discrimination that creates a barrier to care. The ICN (2001b) urges its national member associations to:

> actively participate in sensitising and educating the public about HIV/AIDS; take measures to combat violence against women including rape, sexual abuse, child prostitution and trafficking; work to protect the basic human rights of people living with HIV/AIDS, their families, the public and nurses who care for those living with HIV/AIDS.

The Canadian Association of Nurses in AIDS Care (2000) has called for more specialist training for nurses to respond to the specific needs of HIV/AIDS patients. The association pointed out that care for HIV/AIDS patients requires in-depth knowledge of disease prevention, health promotion, harm reduction and palliative care.

According to UNAIDS, injecting drug use is one of the primary causes of HIV transmission in Europe and Central Asia, where it is responsible for 80% of all HIV cases. Despite these figures, very little is being done to provide access to clean needles, sterilising materials, or drop-off points for used needles. Such measures are recommended by UNAIDS (2005b) to combat the spread of the

---

* A range of UN documents on HIV are available at http://www.ohchr.org/english/issues/hiv/document.htm; Human Rights Watch publications on HIV/AIDS and human rights are available at: http://hrw.org/doc/?t=hivaids_pub.

disease. One NGO report concluded that attempts by Russia and Ukraine to reduce drug use by increasing spending on law enforcement, at the expense of public health policies, was ineffective (Malinowska-Sempruch *et al.* 2003). This is particularly serious since 'the current epidemic in Russia and Ukraine is unique in that the majority of infections continue to be linked to injecting drug use' (p. 12).

The particularities of HIV/AIDS require public health specialists to address issues that formerly remained on the fringes of public health discourse, and which, in many countries, are not the material of daily media discussion. Issues include: ensuring clean needles for drug users; protection of the health of women and men engaged in commercial sex; promotion of safer sexual practices, particularly among adolescent girls. This need extends to high-income countries where rising infection rates among some groups suggest that advances in treatment and care have not been matched by consistent progress in prevention (UN 2006).

Some of this health-promotion work conflicts with laws and practices in many countries. There is also a need for a wider appreciation that ensuring the most effective care for patients requires the protection of carers, educators and human-rights defenders.

CONCLUSION

This chapter has touched on a few of the numerous challenges and opportunities faced by nurses in increasingly globalised health settings. Some of the main issues around nursing, health and human rights are exemplified by three key themes.

- **Ensuring quality of care**. Nurses are key to ensuring that the human right to health is fulfilled, and that care meets basic human rights standards. As a large, organised and well-regulated professional group, nurses are well placed to advocate for human rights at an international, national and local level.
- **Ensuring equitable access to treatment and care**. MDGs and other development and human rights standards aim to ensure that the right to the highest attainable standard of health and access to healthcare is shared by all.
- **Nurse recruitment**. Healthcare providers, while supporting the rights of nurses to seek self-advancement and valuable professional experiences abroad, should encourage nursing practice within the local healthcare system through providing suitable opportunities and incentives for nurses.

Nurses play a key role in maintaining and upholding the right to health. Despite the many pressures globalisation presents to nurses (economic; political), it also offers many opportunities for nurses to use emerging tools, such as improved information and technology, to advance the right to health.

RECOMMENDATIONS

In aiming to enhance the role of nursing in promoting the realisation of the right to health individual nurses could:

- ❐ utilise improvements in global information and communications to share good practice in promoting human rights, especially where innovations have taken place in resource-poor settings.

Nursing organisations could:

- ❐ explicitly acknowledge the link between the work of the nursing profession and the rights of citizens to the highest attainable standard of physical and mental health
- ❐ use a rights-based analysis to frame any submission to government and health funders in support of increased or modified health expenditure or changes to health policy
- ❐ ensure that information on human rights is included in publications directed at nurses and midwives.

Nurse educators could:

- ❐ ensure that the advocacy role of nurses and midwives and the monitoring of human rights violations are addressed in teaching courses
- ❐ develop links with health organisations in order to stimulate and contribute to training and research on subjects such as the effects of economic globalisation on the right to health.

REFERENCES

Amnesty International. Women, HIV/AIDS and Human Rights. London, ACT 77/084/2004. Available at: http://web.amnesty.org/library/Index/ENGACT770842004 (accessed 24 June 2007).

Amnesty International. Human Rights and Privatization. London: AI Index: POL 34/003/2005. Available at: http://web.amnesty.org/library/index/engpol340032005; (accessed 24 June 2007).

Amnesty International. Caring for Human Rights: challenges and opportunities for nurses and midwives. London: Amnesty International; 2006. Available at: http://web.amnesty.org/library/Index/ENGACT750032006 (accessed 24 June 2007).

Beirne M. Social and Economic Rights as Agents for Change. In: Harvey C, editor. Human Rights in the Community: rights as agents for change. London: British Institute of Human Rights; 2005: 43–65.

Canadian Association of Nurses. *Position Statement: recognition of* HIV/AIDS *nursing as a speciality.* Adopted 25 November 2000. AIDS Care. 2000. Available at: http://canac.org/english/PROGRAMS.htm (accessed 24 June 2007).

CEDAW. *Convention on the Elimination of all Forms of Discrimination Against Women.* Adopted by UN General Assembly, resolution 34/180, 18 December 1979. Available at http://www.ohchr.org/english/law/pdf/cedaw.pdf (accessed 24 June 2007).

CEDAW Committee. Committee on the elimination of discrimination against women. General recommendation No. 19, Violence against women. 1992. Available at: http://www2.ohchr.org/english/law/cedaw.htm (accessed 1 May 2008).

Center for Reproductive Law and Policy. *State of Denial: adolescent reproductive rights in Zimbabwe.* New York. 2002. Available at: www.reproductiverights.org/pdf/zimbabwe_report.pdf (accessed 24 June 2007).

CESCR. *General Comment 3, para.* 9. 1990. Available at: http://www.ohchr.org/english/bodies/cescr (accessed 24 June 2007).

CESCR. *General Comment 14 of the Committee on Economic, Social and Cultural Rights.* E/C.12/2004/4, 11 August 2000. Available at: http://www.unhchr.ch/tbs/doc.nsf/(symbol)/E.C.12.2000.4.En (accessed 24 June 2007).

CESCR. *Concluding Observations of the* UN *Committee on Economic, Social and Cultural Rights: the United Kingdom.* E/C/12/1/Add/79, 5 June 2002. Available at: www.unhchr.ch/tbs/doc.nsf/(Symbol)/E.C.12.1.Add.79.En (accessed 24 June 2007).

CRC. *Committee on the Rights of the Child, General Comment 5, para.* 43. CRC/GC/2003/5, 27 November 2003. Available at: http://www.unhchr.ch/tbs/doc.nsf/(symbol)/CRC.GC.2003.5.En (accessed 24 June 2007).

de Mesquita JB, Gordon M. *The International Migration of Health Workers: a human rights analysis.* London. 2005. Available at: http://www.medact.org (accessed 24 June 2007).

Gürsoy E, Vural G. Nurses' and Midwives' Views on Approaches to Hymen Examination. Nursing Ethics. 2003; **10**: 485–96.

ICESCR. *The International Covenant on Economic, Social and Cultural Rights.* Adopted 1966. Available at: http://www.unhchr.ch/html/menu3/b/a_cescr.htm (accessed 24 June 2007).

ICN. *Policy Background Paper on Nursing and Development.* Adopted 2000. Available at: http://www.icn.ch (accessed 24 June 2007).

ICN. *Publicly Funded Accessible Health Care.* Adopted 1995, reviewed 2001a. Available at: http://www.icn.ch (accessed 24 June 2007).

ICN. *Position Statement: Acquired Immunodefiency Syndrome (AIDS).* Adopted 1989, revised 2001b. Available at: http://www.icn.ch/psAIDS00.htm (accessed 24 June 2007).

ICN. *The ICN Code of Ethics for Nurses.* 2006. Available at: http://www.icn.ch/icncode.pdf (accessed 24 June 2007).

Khan I. Secretary-General, Amnesty International. Speech to the XV International Congress on HIV/AIDS, Bangkok, July 2004. Available at: http://www.aidslaw.ca/publications/interfaces/downloadFile.php?ref=844 (accessed 1 May 2008).

Kim J, Motsei M. Women Enjoy Punishment: attitudes and experiences of gender-based violence among PHC nurses in rural South Africa. *Social Science and Medicine.* 2002; **54**: 1243–54.

Malinowska-Sempruch K, Hoover J, Alexandrova A. *Unintended Consequences: drug policies fuel the* HIV *epidemic in Russia and Ukraine.* New York: International Harm Reduction

Development Program Open Society Institute; 2003. Available at: http://www.soros.org/initiatives/ihrd/articles_publications/publications/unintendedconsequences_20030414/unintended_consequences.pdf (accessed 24 June 2007).

McKenzie K. Racism and Health. *British Medical Journal.* 2003; **326**: 65–6.

Muula A, Mfutso-Bengo J, Makoza J. The Ethics of Developed Nations Recruiting from Developing Countries: the case of Malawi. *Nursing Ethics.* 2003; **10**(4): 433–8.

PAHO. *Understanding and Responding to HIV/AIDS-related Stigma and Discrimination in the Health Sector.* Washington DC: PAHO; 2003. p. 7. Available at: www.paho.org/English/AD/FCH/AI/stigma-l.htm (accessed 24 June 2007).

Smedley BD, Stith AY, Nelson AR, editors. Unequal Treatment: confronting racial and ethnic disparities in health care. Washington DC: National Academies Press; 2003.

South Africa. *Constitution of the Republic of South Africa.* 1996: ch. 2, sect. 27. Available at: http://www.polity.org.za/html/govdocs/constitution/saconst.html (accessed June 2007).

Surlis S, Hyde A. HIV-positive Patients Experiences of Stigma During Hospitalisation. *Journal of the Association of Nurses in AIDS Care.* 2001; **12**: 68–77.

UN. *Millennium Declaration.* UN General Assembly Resolution. A/RES/55/2. 2000. Available at: www.un.org/millennium/declaration/ares552e.htm (accessed 24 June 2007).

UN. *Millennium Development Goals.* 2001. Available at: http://www.un.org/millenniumgoals/ (accessed 24 June 2007).

UN. *The Millennium Development Goals Report.* 2006. Available at: http://mdgs.un.org/unsd/mdg/Resources/Static/Products/Progress2006/MDGReport2006.pdf (accessed 2 July 2007).

UNAIDS. *HIV-related Stigma, Discrimination and Human Rights Violations: case studies of successful programmes.* Geneva: UNAIDS; 2005a. Available at: http://data.unaids.org/publications/irc-pub06/JC999-HumRightsViol_en.pdf (accessed 28 June 2007).

UNAIDS. *Joint UNAIDS Statement on HIV Prevention and Strategies for Drug Users.* 2005b. Available at http://www.unaids.org (accessed 24 June 2007).

WHO. *25 Questions & Answers on Health and Human Rights.* Geneva: WHO; 2002a. p. 10. Available at: http://www.who.int/hhr/en/ (accessed 24 June 2007).

WHO. *Strategic Directions for Strengthening Nursing and Midwifery Services.* Geneva: WHO; 2002b. Available at: http://www.who.int/health-services-delivery/nursing/ (accessed 24 June 2007).

7

Ethical ambiguity: can one do 'right' in a 'wrong' situation? The case of Machsomwatch

Nurith Wagner

INTRODUCTION

Terrorism is a global threat. Do we have the right to prevent terror by all means, even those that include infringement of basic human rights?

Terror attacks have resulted in hundreds of deaths and thousands of severely wounded people, and created genuine fear and a deep feeling of insecurity among Israeli people, leading to a policy of erecting barriers, checkpoints and fences. These checkpoints impede movement from village to village, from village to town, and are mainly inside Palestinian territory, not controlling entry into Israel. The checkpoints are officially intended to prevent terrorist movements and thus terror attacks.

Machsomwatch (Checkpoint watch) (MW) was founded in 2001 by three Israeli women following media reports of violations of human rights of Palestinians transiting Israeli Defence Forces (IDF) and Border Police checkpoints (CPs) in the West Bank and Jerusalem. Every day women go out to some 40 CPs in two shifts.

The second Intifada (the resistance by Palestinians against Israeli occupation starting in 2000 and effectively still ongoing) has produced startling statistics: 5000 Israelis wounded in terror attacks between the years 2000 and 2005. They were people riding on a bus, sitting in a restaurant, shopping in a mall. Many more Palestinians were killed and injured during the same time. During that period, I was the Director of Nursing at Hadassah Medical Center, where we cared for about 2500 people, or about half of the wounded.

Terror attacks resulted in genuine fear and deep feelings of insecurity on the Israeli side, which eventually led to the policy of barriers, CPs and fences. The intended effects of the CPs were:

❑ more security and protection for the Israeli population
❑ apprehension of terrorists.

The unintended effects were:
❑ the restriction of movement and control in matters of everyday life of the Palestinian population, resulting in an immeasurable increase in frustration and hate
❑ in Israel, an equally immeasurable impact on the 'souls' of young Israeli soldiers and the collective ethic of Israeli society.

In this chapter I will share some of the major dilemmas that are embedded in the activities at the CPs from my personal viewpoint as an Israeli woman, a nurse, a mother, and the mother of a soldier, and a member of MW. The dilemmas faced, put in the form of questions throughout this text, are described through incidences while on duty as a MW member. All the women of MW grapple with these dilemmas between personal and professional values and beliefs, and the duty to respect universal human rights: can one do 'right' in a 'wrong' situation?

MACHSOMWATCH

The organisation numbers close to 500 women from all over Israel, all of them volunteers. Each day two shifts (morning and afternoon) go out to some 40 CPs and barriers, mainly those within the West Bank. These CPs impede movement from village to village, from village to town, and are inside Palestinian territory. They are not controlling entry to Israel; they are officially intended to prevent terrorist movement and thereby terror attacks.

The MW activity aims to:
❑ protest against the occupation and the existence of the CPs
❑ witness and report on a website any unacceptable behaviour by soldiers towards Palestinians and human rights violations such as intimidation and restrictions on movement
❑ intervene (where and when possible) and offer help in humanitarian-related events
❑ improve physical and other conditions at the CPs.

I will describe some of my group's experiences at Hawarra CP. Hawarra is a small town not far from Nablus (a large city run by the Palestinian Authority), which Israelis are not allowed to enter. Hawarra is the biggest CP in the West Bank and serves an average of 6000 persons daily. Ambulances are allowed to cross the CP after checking, supposedly without delay; trucks can unload at a back-to-back area on a road nearby. A small market selling drinks and food has formed near the CP, which closes at midnight.

Tuesday morning is my shift, together with two other women. We drive through a beautiful landscape of ancient olive trees, old Arab villages and Israeli settlements side by side with fences dividing them. On our drive towards Hawarra, which is a permanent CP, there are also temporary CPs, fences across the road and around the Arab villages, all for security reasons, making the lives of Palestinians very difficult. They cannot move freely in their own territories, get to work, to their olive trees, to school, hospital, or to a doctor's clinic, or just to meet relatives or friends, without special permits.

On our way to the Hawarra CP we stop at one of the many temporary check-points, Tapuach CP. We count the cars waiting to get through. When we see that there are detained people, we inquire what the reason is, and in humanitarian cases, we first talk with the commander at the CP and then, if needed, we call different people from a contact list: the army, the Israeli District Coordinating Office (DCO), Ministry of Health, journalists and others who have the authority, or the will, to help in humanitarian cases (death in the family or very old or ill people). We have our MW tags on and our car is marked, too, so the Palestinians and the soldiers can recognise us.

A Palestinian man waiting in line in his car waves towards us and begs us to stay at the CP: 'Just by you being there', he says, 'the waiting time is shortened.' More than 30 cars wait in line at the CP. The Israeli cars pass without having to stop. There is a woman sitting in a cab with her husband, her mother and her 5-year-old son. The woman looks sick, pale, in pain from gallbladder complications. The family is on its way to Mukassed Hospital in south Jerusalem, but the cab does not have a permit to drive into Israel. We stop another car, and help the woman, her mother and son in. The husband is not permitted to accompany his wife. They drive away. We call our contacts and, after an hour, the husband leaves for Jerusalem to be with his wife.

Ten minutes later we drive through the village of Hawarra and to the CP. On our arrival at the Hawarra CP, we find a crowd of Palestinians trying to get into Nablus. There are three lines of people waiting: one line for women and children, one for old people and one for the young. Young people are considered potential terrorists; the age is defined daily either as between 16 and 36 or as between 20 and 35. Palestinians have to get a special passing permit with the ID card at the DCO office. The long and nerve-racking waits are a clear reason for the distress and tension at the CP. After passing one CP people will be halted and checked again and again at other CPs, and each time there is waiting in line so that documentation can be checked. The rules at the CPs change every day, based on intelligence information about terrorist threats. The Palestinians never know if they will be able to get to their destination.

THE FIRST QUESTION

Is the restriction on the Palestinian population movement justifiable as a means of preventing suicidal terror attacks? Can we balance our need for security and the Palestinians' rights to free movement?

The ICN *Code of Ethics for Nurses* (ICN 2000) states in the preamble that 'Inherent in nursing is respect for human rights'. Conflict arises when my rights clash with the rights of another. The prevailing assumption is that our safety comes first, and that the CPs prevent terror attacks and are therefore justified. Even if we accept this assumption, which most of the MW women do not, we argue that one cannot measure the growing hatred and frustration fed by the daily waiting at the CPs and its effects. Because of the occurrence of so many suicide bomb attacks by Palestinians, we Israelis tend to generalise and view Palestinians collectively as dangerous. Many Israelis had hoped that the Palestinians would take action against terrorist and suicide attacks, especially since they caused the Palestinian population so much suffering, but this hope did not materialise. The Palestinians either did not want, or were not able to prevent terror. Many of them view terror as a justified means to fight the occupation. While we do not agree with this view, the question remains on how we can balance our need for security with the Palestinians' needs and basic human rights (Lacopino 1995; Toebes 1999; Tomasevski 1995).

THE SECOND QUESTION

How can we empathise with the young soldiers who are doing a job that they were sent to do by our own democratically elected government, and at the same time empathise with the suffering of the Palestinians?

At the Hawarra CP there was terrible tension. The soldiers were nervous and under a lot of pressure. The day before, a 16-year-old Palestinian boy was caught with an explosives belt. The soldiers themselves are just kids, frightened, and most of them dislike being at the CPs. Then, here come these MW women, many of them looking like their grandmothers, and watch, criticise and inform about their behaviour or misbehaviour, on their Internet site. Most of the soldiers are good young kids, but being in this situation for months changes them and they become cynical, lose their compassion and become task oriented: preventing terrorists from passing at any price, catching the bad guys and watching for their own safety first. In all honesty, as a mother, I would also tell my son to look after his own safety first. Soldiers have been shot, stabbed or blown up at the CPs.

Our relationship with the soldiers is usually good, but it is also ambivalent. The army recognises us; officers meet with us, read our reports and react. They are not always happy with what is published and complain that it is one-sided, and that we care only about the Palestinians' rights and forget that the soldiers are endangering their own lives. We remind them that since we, the Israelis, are in control, it is our responsibility to ensure the Palestinians' basic human rights, especially their right to healthcare. The monitoring we do at the CPs has an effect, even when it is not appreciated by everyone. We always intervene through the commander first and only when not successful do we then go to our other contacts.

On another Tuesday, a young Palestinian, about 17 years old, was handcuffed, blindfolded and ordered to sit on the floor. He was frightened and cried. We tried to understand why he was detained and the soldiers said that he was connected to terrorism, and they were holding him until the army police could interrogate him. Later, I had a talk with one of the soldiers, who asked me why I am at the CP and if my children were in the army. He was surprised to learn that my son is a colonel in the air force. He told me that he had not asked to be on duty at the CP. At the beginning he had considered the Palestinians as people and saw older persons as his grandparents, but being there for three months had changed him. He is doing his job by looking out for the safety of his comrades and by preventing terror attacks. He is counting the days until he finishes his army duty.

Our relationship with the Palestinians is ambiguous. Quite often, when Palestinians thank us, even when we are not able to help them, I feel upset and frustrated. However, I remind myself that on our shifts we do manage to bring some measure of humane judgement into the frequently changing rules and interpretations of the rules. Sometimes our mere presence stops the soldiers from delaying dozens of people and cars for long hours for no operational reason. We try to shorten the Palestinians' waiting time and restore at least some of their human dignity. Once, when we were not able to help, a Palestinian man asked if we just come to watch their suffering. We explained that we try to help, but are not able to do so in all cases.

THE THIRD QUESTION

Can we protect Israeli citizens without humiliating and intimidating other people, and without harming the sick?

Ambulances are always checked at the CPs. This is because in one suicide attack with dozens of casualties, the explosives had been transported in Red Crescent ambulances, and at other times, explosives have been found hidden under stretchers. If ambulances carry sick people, the vehicles are checked, but they are not supposed to wait in line. When there is a prolonged delay, we ask the commander of the CP to do something about it, as the sick, elderly people and infants do not constitute a security risk. The delays at the CP cause people to miss their doctor's appointment, which affects their health. If they go in an ambulance they pass much faster, but many sick Palestinians do not have the money to pay for an ambulance ride and have to walk 500 metres from the taxi rank, wait in the humanitarian line at the CP, and then walk to the taxi rank on the other side. Sometimes, the person accompanying the sick is not allowed to pass. Often the soldiers themselves stop cars at the CP and try to get sick, old and handicapped people a ride to the taxi rank on the other side.

The answer to the third question is that the situation is humiliating and stressful but, if the soldiers have to do the work they are sent to do, they should do it in a polite and efficient way, but even then the situation is harmful to the sick.

THE FOURTH QUESTION

Do we, by intervening in cases of emergency medical care, exclude other basic human rights?

On another shift, a young Israeli Arab woman came with a boy, about four years old; she wanted to go to a village near Nablus to her father's funeral. She came without a passing permit and the soldiers would not let her pass, as Israeli citizens are not permitted to pass. She was very pale. We asked her to sit down, and asked if she had eaten or drank. No, she whispered, it is the Ramadan, and she would not eat or drink. We called the DCO and she was able to pass.

Sometimes, at the end of the day, we return home and report on the Internet that it had been a good day; the soldiers were polite, worked efficiently. Still, the tension, frustration and humiliation are always there. There are doctors, lawyers, nurses and students, standing at the CP and waiting. Medical personnel should not be stopped, but I always feel shame for us and for them, for our role and for theirs, as together we let such an unbearable situation continue. While we are the occupiers, the Palestinians only recently elected a government that is yet unwilling to renounce terror. In this situation we can see that, when we consider preserving life by eliminating terror attacks as the primary right, we place other basic human rights, such as going to a funeral, as secondary.

THE FIFTH QUESTION

Do our interventions to improve the conditions at the CPs countervail our protest against the existence of the CPs?

There is a discussion among MW members about our interventions in the harsh conditions at the CPs: do we jeopardise our goal of fighting against the CPs in the first instance? MW emphasises that our purpose is not to make the occupation and the CP more bearable, but to make Israelis aware of them. At first, the Hawarra CP was without a roof, toilet or running water. The long wait on hot summer days, or on wet, cold and rainy days in the winter was unbearable. On our shifts we shared our water bottles and, after our interventions in 2004, the army built a permanent CP with a roof, with running water and a toilet. A year later the southern CP was closed. The Palestinians can go into Nablus freely, but when returning they are checked and passing takes at least one-and-a-half hours. Revolving gates were installed to control the flow of people and prevent suicide attacks in the CP, but the turnstiles are too narrow, and they become dangerous when the place is packed and people, mainly mothers with children and with parcels, get stuck.

The dilemma raised in question five is not solved. By making improvements at the CPs, we can be seen to be more or less accepting them, which countervails our protest against them; but, at the same time, we cannot stand by and see the suffering without trying to intervene.

THE SIXTH QUESTION

What are the effects of the CPs on our soldiers and on the ethics of Israeli society?

On yet another shift, a 19-year-old female soldier was sitting on the floor crying bitterly. It turned out that this young soldier had asked a Palestinian woman of about her own age who held an infant in her arms to show her ID card. The woman thought the soldier had asked to check the baby and she passed her baby to the soldier. The young soldier was so taken aback by the compliance of the mother, who was ready to give her baby to the soldier, she couldn't stop crying. The soldier refused to return to her duty at the CPs.

Our concern is also for the future of Israeli society, on which the occupation has left its destructive mark. We know that the CP experience of power, control, intimidation, violence, fear and frustration marks our youth, and that it will also have an effect upon their future, as spouses, parents and citizens. Will young soldiers see an abusive or a compassionate face when looking in the mirror?

Two Palestinian women about 30 years of age came to the CP one day while our group was on duty. One woman was legally blind. They explained that they had an appointment with the ophthalmologist in an Israeli settlement. The travel permit was for the day before. The CP commander sent a jeep to the DCO to get the women an entrance permit so that they could enter. We called the doctor, who promised to wait for them, and the permit arrived. The women passed the CP and we hoped that the doctor was still there waiting for them.

CONCLUSION

When we, as peace and human rights activists, watch the soldiers, we consider them as agents of the occupation. We watch them as if they are our children, the next generation of our society, and are appalled by the intolerable experience they undergo and how their moral values become crushed. The policy of oppression and dehumanisation is inherent in the control over other people. It seeps into the consciousness and behaviour of the soldiers serving at CPs and in the occupied territories. This does not comply with the basic Israeli law of human dignity and liberty, which must be a right for all. Those laws do not stop at the borders and young soldiers, who receive legitimisation for assailing human dignity, find it hard to internalise a culture that is grounded in human rights that Israel, as a democratic society, aims to impart.

Our responsibility is to help the Palestinians in cases of emergency. We assist where we can with the immediate need but, in so doing, we neglect the basic human right of access to healthcare in the occupied territories. I know that the restriction of movement on Palestinians has a serious impact on their ability to work, to get to school, and to pursue normal social activity. All this influences their well-being and health. By helping, are we ignoring other needs that are compromised by the CPs? We want the CPs to be removed, but are we indirectly sustaining them by intervening to try to make conditions at them 'humane'?

The intended overall aims of MW are:

◻ to guard respect for the person, and to alleviate the suffering of Palestinians
◻ to raise awareness in Israeli society of the effects of the barriers on Palestinians, as well as on the soldiers.

The unintended outcome of our activities at the CPs may be the 'failure of success': if humanitarian crises are solved, it becomes more acceptable to keep the situation as it is.

While we are doing 'right' in a 'wrong' situation, I have doubts about how effective any such activity is. Yet, our presence at 40 CPs twice a day every day of the year ($40 \times 2 \times 365$) equals 29 200 checkpoint observations per year; this is a considerable commitment and demonstration.

We are caught in the double bind of living in a situation with a traditional enemy who has sworn to eliminate us (and extremists repeating this threat), while we are sworn to prevent this by all means; and 'all means' includes infringement of basic human rights. I also believe that one day the Palestinians will have to face the implications of their choice of struggle, which includes terror and suicide bombings, for their own society.

We know that breaking this vicious cycle is the responsibility of Israelis and Palestinians alike, but we also believe that the rest of the world shares this responsibility. Instead of looking for 'who to blame' and dividing the world into 'good guys' and 'bad guys', the victims and the oppressor, there is a need to grasp and learn to live with the ambiguity of a situation and the double binds in which we all live.

Neither barriers nor borders can stop viruses, hatred, frustration and terror. We live in a global world. We are responsible for one another. We have no future unless we break out of the old world view of 'us' versus 'the enemy'.

Why wait for a global pandemic that kills not only fowl but also millions of people before we work together and find ways for all of us to survive and live our lives in dignity? It seems absurd that only the threat of a global catastrophe should teach us to cooperate and live together.

If we want to break the cycle of suffering of the Palestinians and the Israelis alike, we cannot wait for the world, or governments, to change. We cannot stay in the waiting places. We have to shift our dialogue and our actions from blaming each other to taking responsibility and a stand: enough of bloodshed.

Today we need both bottom-up activities, such as those of the women of MW, as well as top-down political leadership with courage and vision on all sides, foregoing the zero-sum game and seeking win–win situations where all of us have hope for the future.

We owe it to ourselves to be aware. We owe it to our children. We owe to give witness. We owe to show respect and reach out. We owe the Palestinians a fair chance to build their nation state. I cannot speak for what the Palestinians owe themselves, but I do know that the Palestinians owe us a life without fear of being blown up in a bus or a café.

Our reality is complex. Our history is fraught with war and tragedy. We need the 'simple solutions' of respect for the needs of the other. As a street poster I saw in the US said: 'In violence we lose ourselves'.

REFERENCES

ICN. *Code of Ethics for Nurses*. Geneva: ICN; 2000.

Lacopino V. Human rights concerns for the twenty-first century. In: Majumdar SK, *et al.*, editors. *Medicine and Health Care into the Twenty-first Century*. Easton, PA: Pennsylvania Academy of Science; 1995. pp. 376–91.

Toebes B. *The Right to Health as a Human Right in International Law*. Antwerp: Hart Intersentia; 1999.

Tomasevski K. Health Rights. In: Eide A., *et al.*, editors. *Economic, Social and Cultural Rights*. Leiden: Martinus Nijhoff; 1995. pp. 125–42.

Recruitment, migration and regulation

8

Standards of nursing in the era of HIV/AIDS: Tanzania as a case study

Gustav Moyo

INTRODUCTION

Standards in the healthcare services provide boundaries and expectations for practice and describe a level of care, values and priorities that are common to the specialty and to the professions providing that care. Such standards are both ethical and legal requirements that aim to promote quality of care and to protect consumers receiving this service. This chapter focuses on the impact of HIV/AIDS on these standards.

The first cases of HIV/AIDS in Tanzania were reported in 1983 and were experienced then as a new and strange disease. However, now it is viewed and experienced as a common problem, affecting most families. The emergence of the HIV/AIDS pandemic has seriously compromised standards of nursing, as it has increased the morbidity rate of both the population and the nurses, and overstretched available resources that were already in short supply.

African countries south of the Sahara have been heavily affected socially and economically by HIV/AIDS. Since the arrival of this pandemic, we have learned several things. For example, we know that:

1   the majority of in-patients have HIV/AIDS as an underlying problem
2   the epidemic has contributed significantly to the problem of absenteeism among health workers
3   the infected/affected health workers perform sub-optimally for long periods of time, contributing to an increased workload for others
4   highly experienced health workers are lost, as they are dying long before their retirement age
5   much money is lost through lengthy paid sick leave
6   many nurses are lost to the health service as they choose to join less stressful and less risky professions

7 many nurses are lost as they choose to migrate to countries with less HIV/AIDS prevalence.

All these factors make the healthcare that is provided of poorer quality than it would be otherwise. The burden of so many sick people in the healthcare system, combined with the loss of healthcare workers, creates powerful interacting national and regional problems in maintaining healthcare standards.

THE HIV/AIDS PANDEMIC IN SUB-SAHARAN AFRICA: THE LARGER CONTEXT

The term sub-Saharan Africa (SSA) is used to describe the area of the African continent that lies south of the Sahara desert. It includes 42 countries on the mainland and six island countries. Within this area lies the East African Community (EAC), incorporating the countries of Tanzania, Kenya, Uganda, Burundi and Rwanda. This area is famous for its game parks and natural beauty. To an outsider, these countries provide a wonderful place for a holiday of game viewing; however, the HIV/AIDS pandemic has ravaged the people in cities, towns and villages to create serious problems for maintaining healthcare standards in the region.

According to WHO statistics, of the 39.5 million people living with HIV, 24.7 million are in SSA. Of the 4.3 million new infections in 2006, 2.8 million were in this region. However, 2.1 million of the 2.9 million global deaths from AIDS in 2006 were also in SSA. In addition, this area has the highest adult prevalence rate (5.9%) of any region globally. As of June 2006, the estimated number of people with HIV/AIDS receiving treatment in SSA, was 1 040 000, and the number needing treatment was 4 600 000. Worldwide, less than one in five people at risk of becoming infected has access to basic prevention services. Only one in eight people who want to be tested are currently able to do so. This is particularly true in SSA.

In summary, SSA is the most affected region in the world with regard to the HIV/AIDS pandemic. Two-thirds of all people living with HIV live here. Almost three-quarters of all adult and child deaths due to AIDS have occurred in SSA.

EAST AFRICA: THE HIV/AIDS PANDEMIC

While East Africa has a developed tourist business, many people live in grinding poverty, dependent on agriculture for employment and income. Almost half (46.5%) of the people living in the SSA countries survive on less than USD1 per day. Nearly one-third of the children in the region are underweight and under five years of age. This is not a new problem, but one that existed long before the pandemic. The long-established Under Five Clinics throughout the region attest to this fact. Children have been hard hit for many years, and the HIV/AIDS situation simply reinforces this large socio-economic problem. The infant mortality rate remains at 110 death per 1000 live births. The maternal mortality rate or maternal deaths per 100 000 live births stands at 920. What such a figure means in reality is that countries in this region have poor standards of care and have many infants and young children without mothers to care for them. In some cases, care is left to the father or grandparents, or even neighbours, while at other times these children are placed in orphanages because there is no one to care for them.

TANZANIA

The United Republic of Tanzania, which includes the mainland country of Tanzania and the islands of Mafia, Pemba and Zanzibar, is the largest country in East Africa and ranks thirty-first in land mass worldwide. With a population of 39.4 million, it ranks thirty-second worldwide. This area is known for scenery that includes Lakes Victoria, Nyasa and Tanganyika, as well as the highest peak in Africa, Mount Kilimanjaro. The country gained its independence in 1961.

The statistics are similar to those for many developing countries (Central Intelligence Agency (CIA) 2007). Average life expectancy at birth is estimated at approximately 50 years, annual per capita income is less than USD1 per day (USD340 per year), and the literacy rate is 69.4% as of 2007, which is better than in some other countries. More men than women can read and write. The infant mortality rate is 76 per 1000 live births, while the mortality rate for children under five years is 122 per 1000. It is interesting to note that 43.4% of births are attended by skilled health staff. Along with the usual health and health system problems in a country like Tanzania, this situation had been aggravated by the influx of refugees from neighbouring countries such as Burundi, Rwanda, Somalia and the Congo, in addition to the onslaught of HIV/AIDS in the country.

PEOPLE WITH AIDS IN TANZANIA

While the reported data on HIV/AIDS provides information about East Africa in general, the following information is specific to Tanzania. The cumulative total of reported cases since 1983 is 192 532, with 5% of these being people below the age of 15. People in the age range of 20–49 years remained the most affected.

One source of data on HIV/AIDS infection has been from blood donations.

HIV prevalence testing for blood donors in Tanzania in 2004 showed that the average rate of HIV prevalence from 154 045 ppeople who donated blood nationally was 7.7%. Most blood donors were men (83.7%) with a prevalence rate of 7.2% and the rest were women with a prevalence rate of 10.7%. In 2004, nearly two million people were living with HIV in Tanzania, slightly more women than men. The estimated annual deaths in that year from HIV were 187 350.

Management of people with AIDS has created more burdens for an already weak economy. People with an advanced stage of the disease are admitted to hospitals more often and stay longer in hospitals. With the existing total number of beds countrywide being around 29 616, the increased number of clients with HIV and AIDS creates challenges in being fair regarding resource distribution. (Ministry of Health (MOH) 1999).

It is estimated that the HIV infections in rural areas will double by the year 2010. The life expectancy at birth in 2004 was 46.8 years for men and 49.1 years for women, which is a decline from 49 and 51 respectively in 1998.

CASE STUDY: AMANA HOSPITAL, DAR ES SALAAM

Amana Hospital lies in Ilala Municipality, and is the only hospital owned by Ilala Municipal Council. Ilala is one of three districts in Dar es Salaam, representing the downtown area. Listing the five causes of death at Amana Hospital gives a snapshot of the disease burden of this East African country.

TABLE 8.1 Causes of death, Amana Hospital

Below 5 years	No.	%	5 years and above	No.	%
Malaria	132	47.6	HIV/AIDS	284	51.0
Pneumonia	93	33.5	Malaria	130	23.3
Anaemia	29	10.4	Tuberculosis	89	16.0
HIV/AIDS	12	4.3	Pneumonia	38	6.8
Tuberculosis	11	3.9	Anaemia	15	2.6
Total	**277**	**100.0**	**Total**	**556**	**100.0**

In Ilala district, there are an estimated 66 000 people living with HIV; 70% of these are within the 20–49 age group. Of 4234 blood donors between July and December 2005, 374 (8.8%) were HIV positive. Of 7555 clients who came for Voluntary Counselling Testing services for HIV, 2224 (29.4%) were HIV positive. This shows that the problem of HIV/AIDS is very high in this district (Ministry of Health and Social Welfare (MOHSW) 2006).

Statistics from the neighbouring district of Temeke presents another grim picture. Its municipal hospital's labour ward has a complement of only 24 midwives, of whom five are normally on duty per eight-hour shift. They deliver an average of 16 babies per shift, with only two delivery beds (MOHSW 2006).

THE WORKFORCE

Various government initiatives have signified challenges to the workforce. One of them, the National HIV/AIDS Care and Treatment Plan was approved by the Cabinet in October 2003 (Government of Tanzania 2003). The plan aims to cover between 400 000 and 500 000 HIV-infected Tanzanians with Anti-Retroviral Therapy (ART) in the period to 2008. The targeted number of patients to be on ART during the first year was about 44 000. This can be achieved only if large numbers of people are counselled, tested and managed. This inevitably means more responsibilities for an already overstretched workforce, which is likely to compromise the quality of care.

Healthcare providers are stigmatised because they work with HIV-positive patients, and without appropriate facilities and protective equipment. They deal with the public's attitudes and perceptions that treating or taking care of people with HIV/AIDS is pointless, since they are incurable. Such attitudes demoralise healthcare workers and push them away from the profession.

A further challenge is the increased occupational exposure of healthcare workers from needle-stick injuries, though accurate data are lacking. In a study conducted on occupational exposure to the risk of HIV infection among health workers in the Mwanza region of Tanzania, it was revealed that 9.2% of 623 nurses and 1.3% of 118 doctors interviewed had pricked themselves (Gumodoka et al. 1997). The study also showed that 22% of nurses working in labour wards and 25% of those working in operating theatres had pricked themselves in the previous months. With the existing HIV prevalence in this region, this shows further areas of vulnerability for nurses.

THE DIVISION OF NURSING SERVICE OF TANZANIA SURVEY

A large number of health workers (232) died before reaching the voluntary retirement age. The years of productivity lost per person ranged from 1 to 29, with an average of 14.3 years. Female nurses and midwives died at younger ages and lost more years of productivity than male nurses. Some regions lost more younger health workers than others. Although the cause of death is usually not revealed, the questioners collected other data that strongly suggested HIV as the cause of death (Annual Regional Nursing Officers Meeting 2006).

TABLE 8.2 Approved and actually filled staff positions for selected cadres of health workers for the years of study

Cadre	2000		2001		2002		2003		2004	
	Approved	Filled	Approved	Filled	Approved	Filled	Approved	Filled	Approved	Filled
Medical Officer	211	94	212	84	215	85	219	87	232	108
Assistant Medical Officer	338	146	341	158	352	184	358	205	379	225
Clinical Officer/ Clinical Assistant	399	327	415	318	397	313	383	334	383	394
Nurse	2703	1814	2770	1435	2812	1524	2762	1638	2713	1946
Lab. Technician	195	122	197	118	205	127	206	141	211	151
Ancillary staff	2147	2056	1821	1990	1822	1891	1852	1876	1850	2066

Among the health workers who died, 170 (67.7%) were known or believed to have been suffering from HIV/AIDS. The designations of the health workers who were believed to have died of HIV/AIDS are:

☐ Medical attendants   66   76.7%
☐ Nurses   48   53.4%
☐ Clinicians   17   51.5%

Equally drastic are the outcomes that impact standards of care in a major way:

> The workers who suffered from HIV/AIDS had been in poor health for between one and 60 months, with an average of 12.6 months. At the time of the study, 55.3% of the health workers who died had not been replaced. Of those not replaced 44.4% were nurses, and 42% were from other clinical categories (Annual Regional Nursing Officers Meeting 2006).

Table 8.2 shows graphically that, in all professional and trained workforce categories, places were not filled, mainly due to bureaucratic difficulties in finding replacements. Numbers of untrained staff, however, have constantly increased, as they are used to replace professional staff. While this means employment opportunities for low or unskilled people, the care given to and received by patients cannot be optimal. Untrained people may not be able to recognise critical signs of illness or cope with emergencies, thus increasing morbidity and mortality among staff and patients. It seems to be a vicious cycle without any hope of breaking out of it.

CONCLUSION

The HIV/AIDS pandemic has hit Africa most severely. The reasons for this are not always clear, but mismanagement, poverty and the consequences of debt in African countries have significantly contributed to a worsening of the situation in all areas of healthcare. This is specifically true for East African countries, but similar situations apply in other sub-Saharan countries, and by extension, other developing countries.

Nurses and many other qualified healthcare staff have migrated to more lucrative situations in Western countries, putting more work and burdens on those left behind. The fact that staff vacancies are not filled may be due not only to migration, but also to inadequate resources to finance the posts. Whatever the reasons, patients inevitably suffer, and the health of the nations concerned is not improving, let alone maintained. The burden on nurses themselves is not only an increased workload, but also knowing that their work is not adequate, leading to demoralisation and even less willingness to care. The effect on patients is inevitably negative, with morbidity and mortality rates increasing across the board.

While nurses who are educated are leaving their jobs, the return on their investment is wasted. Nurses who have migrated may not be happy in their new countries and positions, which may not increase the adoptive countries' results either. What meagre resources are available in Tanzania and other similar countries have been overstretched, leading to poor standards of nursing. This is but one case study, reflecting the realities for all developing countries affected by the HIV/AIDS pandemic.

It is this recognition that is increasingly crucial to all healthcare. The Millenium Development Goals have contributed to some extent to reverse the situation but, until international financial institutions take realistic steps to implement the goals, the detrimental conditions will negate countries' efforts to improve health standards. Nurses themselves, however, need to make the conditions known to their governments, and do everything in their power to reverse the lamentable statistics presented in this chapter.

REFERENCES

Annual Regional Nursing Officers Meeting, Tanzania. Report 2006.

CIA. *The World Factbook. Tanzania.* Available at: https://www.cia.gov/library/publications/the-world-factbook/geos/tz.html (accessed 12 November 2007).

Government of Tanzania. *National HIV/AIDS Care and Treatment Plan.* October 2003. Available at: http://www.districthealthservice.com/cms/upload/policycat_35_9804.pdf (accessed 20 September 2007).

Gumodoka B, Favot I, Berege ZA, Dolmans WMV. Occupational Exposure to the Risk of HIV Infection Among Health Care Workers in Mwanza Region, United Republic of Tanzania. *Bulletin of* WHO. 1997; **75**(2): 133–40.

MOH, Tanzania. *Health Statistics Abstract, Dar es Salaam.* June 1998 and November 1999. Available at: http://www.moh.go.tz/Health%20Indicators.php (accessed 20 September 2007).

MOHSW, Tanzania. *Annual Health Statistical Abstract,* April 2006. (Health report, Ilala Municipality, for six months July–December 2005.)

9

Nurse migration: the donor perspective

Tova Hendel

INTRODUCTION

Globalisation is a broad term used to refer to international economic expansion, as well as to the interdependent economic, political and social processes that accompany the flow of people, capital, goods, information, concepts, images, ideas and values across increasingly diffuse borders and boundaries. Globalisation is more than the internationalisation of commerce and manufacturing. It represents a new development paradigm, creating new links among corporations, international organisations, governments, communities, professionals and families. Globalisation tends to homogenise social, economic and cultural processes. The domination of the free-market ideology that has accompanied globalisation has resulted in both increasing interdependency among local and national economies, and increasing economic vulnerability and instability. Countries are affected in different ways by globalisation, depending on their histories, traditions, cultures and priorities (DeAnne & Hilfinger 2001; Waters 2001; Herdman 2004).

Migration is affected by globalisation and although not new, it is changing as the 'global village' expands. Migration has become increasingly widespread over the past century, motivated by political, economic, psychological and ideological factors. Although immigration aims at improving the immigrants' well-being, it is liable to have profound stress-precipitating, hence maladjustive, consequences (Ben-Sira 1997).

The increasing globalisation of the market has influenced global health, the nursing profession and the nursing workforce. Health is a global concern and nursing is a global profession (OiSaeng 2003). Nursing today operates within the context of a capitalist world economy in which the rapid acceleration of the effects of globalisation cannot be ignored. The flow of internationally educated nurses has increased in tandem with the globalisation processes.

Two common underling assumptions are related to nurse migration:

◻ international nurse migration is natural and is expected to intensify (Aiken *et al.* 2004; Kline 2003; Ross *et al.* 2005)

◻ migration flow patterns largely occur from developing to developed countries (McElmurray *et al.* 2006).

In this chapter, I will examine nurse migration from the point of view of a donor (source) developed country, emphasising factors that may simultaneously influence migration.

REASONS FOR NURSE MIGRATION

Since the late 1980s, a 'globalisation orthodoxy' has emerged, synthesising specific themes imperative for nurses to understand. It is generally accepted that globalisation blurs national boundaries, as governments lose some degree of sovereignty over policy and multinational corporations become increasingly independent (Herdman 2004). In such a climate, the nursing world has become closer and migration of nurses is now common (Seloilwe 2005). The current severe nursing shortage has led to a marked growth in the economic and social migration of nurses. An increasing demand for nurses and a decreasing supply has resulted in heightened competition for the human nursing resource. Nurses move between developing and developed countries, from one developed country to another and between developing countries in the same geographical region. They are now seen as a global workforce of international significance rather than solely the concern of individual nations (Aiken *et al.* 2004; Gerrish 2004; Kingma 2004).

The import of nursing labour and skills to the developed world has become the new trend, whereas in the past, skilled labour came only from the developed world (Seloilwe 2005). This facilitates the mass migration of nurses, as they are actively recruited from the developing world to the West.

Extensive literature on migration exists, pointing out this complex issue, influenced by international, national and individual factors. The empirical literature has demonstrated that factors such as relative income, income inequality, unemployment rates, political and social freedoms are important determinants of migration. Hatton and Williamson (1998) grouped determinants into four categories:

1 wage differentials
2 poverty constraint on movement
3 age profile of populations
4 size of the existing émigré population in the receiving country.

Although the conventional migration theory suggests that individuals migrate to exploit wage differentials, these other components may influence the decision. Nurse migration is also motivated by the search for professional development, better quality of life and personal safety. Pay and learning opportunities continue to be the most frequently reported incentives for nurse migration, especially by nurses from less-developed countries. Career opportunities are considered key incentives for nurses emigrating from high-income countries (Kingma 2001; McElmurray *et al.* 2006; Ross *et al.* 2005). Linda Aiken *et al.* (2004) describe several factors promoting nurse migration: poor wages, economic instability, poorly funded healthcare systems, safety concerns (motivated by circumstances within the health sector or the external environment), and the burdens and risks of AIDS. High levels of nurse burn-out, dissatisfaction and turnover were also found to be factors for nurse migration.

The Philippines, with the support of its government, is a leading primary source country for nurse migration (Aiken *et al.* 2004). There is no other country that produces more nurses than are needed in its own healthcare system, at a level of education that meets the requirements of developed countries. Other primary donor countries are Australia, Canada, South Africa, the UK, China and India (Kline 2003). The US, UK and Canada are leading recipient countries. Data on the actual numbers of nurses entering the US and Canada each year are unavailable. Recruitment to the US, UK and Canada has accelerated since the late 1990s, through the efforts of a rapidly growing number of private recruiting agencies acting as agents for employers seeking nurses internationally to fill growing domestic vacancies (Aiken *et al.* 2004; Ross *et al.* 2005).

The accelerating nurse migration process has fuelled the debate about the consequences for source (donor) and recipient (host) countries, and raises ethical dilemmas. The negative effects of nurse migration from developing countries has created great inequities in overall health conditions between source and recipient countries, widening the gap between them. Migration of nurses from donor countries can create hardships in donor countries, owing to the loss of skilled personnel and weakening of the country's health system, resulting in increased care demands on the nurses who remain and their inability to meet the needs of patients in understaffed organisations (Little 2007).

NURSE MIGRATION INTO AND OUT OF ISRAEL

Israel is a country made up of immigrants from almost every country in the world, comprising a mosaic of people from different religious and cultural backgrounds. Their different ethnic backgrounds and cultures have blended into a melting pot of Israeli life. Each community, however, proudly keeps its traditions alive. Since

1989, a large community (about 1 200 000 people) from the former Soviet Union (FSU) has immigrated to Israel, increasing the Israeli population by approximately 20%. About seven million people live in Israel today; almost 80% are Jews, and the remaining 20% are Muslims and Christians.

In spite of limited resources, many efforts are made to help the new immigrants to adjust to life in their new country. The 1950 Law of Return serves as the legal framework for immigrant absorption in Israel. This law entitles any Jew, except for one who acts against the Jewish people or is a public health or security risk, to settle in Israel. Since the establishment of the State of Israel, the immigrant absorption policy had been one of strong government intervention. Since 1990, the Israeli government has advocated a 'free-market' ideology, implementing it through two major mechanisms: 'direct absorption' and the 'absorption basket'.

Direct absorption means that, on arrival, immigrants are taken to their new homes without first living in transitional accommodation. The absorption basket is a package of services, allowances and entitlements used by immigrants for whatever they choose. After 15 years of this immigration policy there is less government intervention due to immigrants' networks taking the place of government aid (Horowitz 2005).

The Ministry of Immigrant Absorption is responsible for providing government assistance to new immigrants from first setting foot in the country to their integration into every area of life in Israeli society. The Ministry is committed to providing new immigrants with assistance, support and attention, and is motivated by the understanding that ensuring successful absorption will positively impact on the future of Israeli society (Ministry of Immigration Absorption 2007).

Many health professionals have immigrated to Israel since the 1990s, significantly increasing the numbers of physicians and nurses. However, because of the differences in curricula, standards and demands required, the Ministry of Health developed and conducted many courses over the years to enable professional immigrants to meet the new requirements and integrate into the various health organisations.

The country's population is served by an extensive health network comprising hospitals, clinics and mother-and-child care centres, offering state-of-the-art healthcare by highly qualified physicians, nurses and other healthcare professionals. Our high-quality health services, together with the Center for International Cooperation of the Ministry of Foreign Affairs, enables us to host and train thousands of health professionals from many countries, including our Arab neighbours and the Palestinian Authority in Gaza and Jericho. The aims of these programmes are to provide the trainees with the opportunity to enhance their professional capabilities, develop professional leadership skills and learn from each other. The programmes take place at acute-care hospitals, children's medical centres, community health services, family health centres and rehabilitation centres.

THE NURSING WORKFORCE

The total number of nurses in Israel at the end of 2006 was 53 572, including 37 962 (71%) registered nurses and 15 610 (29%) practical nurses. Nurses up to the age of 60 (41 355) at the end of 2006 comprised 30,790 (74%) registered nurses and 10,565 (26%) practical nurses.

The nurse ratio in 2006 was 5.8 per 1000 people, of which 4.3 were registered nurses. Twenty-five per cent of the registered nurses have a BA degree in nursing and 41% have taken a one-year, post-basic course in a sub-specialty, such as midwifery, operating room, oncology, psychiatry, intensive care, community nursing, and so on. About 1200 new registered nurses enter the labour market each year (MOH, Nursing Division 2006).

In Israel, as in many other countries, there is a shortage of nurses. Orly Rotem-Picker and Orly Toren (2005) described several reasons for the shortage of nurses in Israel, including the decrease in numbers of immigrants to Israel since the late 1990s, and nurse migration from Israel. Nurse migration from Israel has been reported in the media, emphasising the growing numbers of nurses intending to emigrate. Foreign nurses who are not permanent residents or citizens are not allowed to work as nurses in Israel.

NURSING EDUCATION: FINANCIAL ASSISTANCE TO MIGRANT NURSING STUDENTS

Nursing education in Israel is largely financed by students and their families, which is a financial hardship for many applicants. The student nursing population reflects the social and cultural pluralism of Israeli society. About 30–35% of the nursing students immigrated as young children with their families from the FSU in the early 1990s, forming a group that comprises about 20% of the total population. An extensive investment is expended on immigrant students. The universities are committed to providing these students with assistance and support during the four years of their professional socialisation process, individually and in groups, helping them to adjust to the new culture and new environment, and successfully finishing their studies.

Immigrant students who have been accepted as regular students at institutions of higher education are eligible for Student Authority assistance from the university. The period of eligibility for Student Authority assistance is 7.5 years from the date of immigration. This period of eligibility may be extended for several reasons, including army service. The Student Authority offers tuition grants for up to three years for undergraduate studies, including a pre-academic programme, and/or for graduate studies, including a supplementary year, if required. This grant is for tuition fees only, and is not dependent on the student's financial or family situation. Additionally, grants are available from other sources. Many of the graduates of the four-year baccalaureate programme continue their studies in post-basic specialisation courses, mainly intensive care unit (ICU) and operating room (OR) courses. A high demand exists for these courses, with a limited number of available places.

NURSE MIGRATION FROM ISRAEL: CAUSES AND IMPACTS

Nurse migration from Israel is part of an international phenomenon that appears to be increasing. Although, according to WHO, Israel is not considered a donor country compared with other countries (Kline 2003), the problem of outflow, even though relatively small, is still worrying. Nurses wishing to emigrate apply to their universities with application forms from abroad to receive confirmation of their studies.

Solid data are lacking concerning the scope of nurse migration patterns. The Nursing Division of the MOH (2006) reported that 1250 nurses asked for application forms for working permits between the years 2002–2006 (24.7% of the total 5049 registered nurses who graduated during these years). Since 2001, 870 nursing students graduated from the BA programme of Tel Aviv University. About 140 application forms were approved during this period, mainly to the US and Canada (about 16%). Figures reflect that most of the graduates (60–70%) wishing to emigrate are former immigrants from FSU.

A wide range of factors contributes to nurse migration, including political, economic, social, legal, historical, cultural and educational ones (Kline 2003; Dovlo 2007; Little 2007). Nurse migration from Israel is part of a wide process of the 'brain drain'. This problem has been examined from sociological and psychological perspectives, exploring personality, demographic and economic factors related to the issue (Adir 1995). Overall, the results suggested that financial and professional incentives, as well as socio-cultural factors, were better predictors and more powerful motivators than personality factors in the decision to emigrate.

According to research data published in 2006 by the Shalem Center, Institute for Economic and Social Policy (Gould & Moav 2006), those with a higher education (BA degree and higher), had a greater tendency to emigrate than those with less education. Among highly educated immigrants in the 25–40 age group, approximately 4.65% left the country during 1995–2002, compared with about 2% with a lower education. The study classified emigrants according to education, employment, income, family status, and number of years in the country. The findings showed that immigrants were not a representative sample of the population. The proportion of well-educated individuals among these emigrants is significantly greater than the proportion in the overall population. The findings are particularly worrisome with respect to immigrants from the FSU. Many educated young people from this group have emigrated to the West. It is estimated that the outflow of Israeli academics, many having no intention of returning, is expected to continue to rise.

Thus far there have been no research studies conducted in Israel to identify and analyse nurse migration. I would like to suggest three main possible influencing factors that may explain this specific socio-political phenomenon.

Immigration from the FSU since 1989

Russian immigrants as a group represent a large minority of the Israeli population (about 16%), and live in a well-established subculture. Successful integration of immigrants in Israel is generally measured by objective parameters, such as work, living conditions, language acquisition and social network. Adaptation, as measured by these parameters, has been found to be positively associated with length of time since arrival here. Distress inherent in the immigration process is not only influenced by the passing of time but also moderated by other factors. These include adverse post-migration conditions to which immigrants may be more vulnerable, personal and social resources, and the ideological motivation and level of commitment to the new society. Socio-demographic characteristics, such as age or gender, may affect the occurrence and experience of stress, as may the availability of personal and social resources (Ben-Sira 1997; Lerner et al. 2005).

Israel's immigration policy differs from that of other migrant societies (e.g. US, Canada, and Australia), which control immigration by establishing priorities, preferences, quotas and other means of limiting immigrant entry. Since its founding, the State of Israel has practised an 'open door' policy for accepting all Jews (but only Jews) who want to settle here. The State views Jewish migration as a returning diaspora, and sees it as the natural right of all Jews to return to their historic homeland. The centrepiece of Israel's religion-based immigration policy is the Law of Return. Jews who immigrate to Israel acquire Israeli citizenship on arrival and are entitled to all benefits conferred by this status. Employment, language learning and social absorption are regarded as interwoven, and actions are undertaken by the government in these realms to facilitate the absorption goals. For many who wanted to leave the FSU, this was the only fast solution, although not always the preferred one (Lewin-Epstein et al. 2003).

Several studies were carried out between 1995 and 2005 aimed at exploring the process of immigrant absorption from psychological and socio-economic aspects. These studies showed that, among immigrants from the FSU, impressive positive changes in objective parameters of adaptation, such as employment, housing conditions and acquisition of host language, had taken place five years after immigration as compared with the first year. However, there was little change in subjective indicators of adaptation, such as satisfaction with living in Israel and perceived social support. After five years in Israel, the psychological distress of the immigrants from the FSU remained high, even though a process of objective adaptation had taken place. Lack of perceived social support, poor family functioning and non-identification with the host society remain important factors related to psychological distress. Feelings of being uprooted and alienated appear to be long-lasting. Education was not found to be a protective factor for distress (Beenstock & Ben-Menahem 1997; Lerner *et al.* 2005). These findings may be one explanation for the emigration of nurses from Israel.

Instability of the political situation

An association exists between political instability and migration. Looking for peace and security is one of the reasons professionals choose to leave their country.

Having being exposed to the violence of the conflict in the region over many years, and experiencing continuous terror attacks directed against the civilian population and military targets, the Israeli public is constantly on the alert. Everyone remembers the national and regional states of emergencies, when normal life routine changed overnight, the heavy damage caused by bombs creating distress and anxiety among the population, a threat to survival, and a fear of the unknown (Hendel *et al.* 2000).

These events are closely followed in the media, with reporting often being a vicarious form of intense emotional involvement in the events. The disruption of daily routine and the exposure of the individual to stressful conditions disrupts the homeostatic resting state and engenders a state of flux, triggering a series of responses intended to enable the organism to adjust to the (altered) prevailing conditions and re-establish homeostasis (Kaplan *et al.* 2005; Shalev *et al.* 2006). Although much appears to hinge on individual factors and psycho-social and societal factors, Zeev Kaplan *et al.* (2005) found that the overall incidence of acute stress symptoms among populations all over the country was high. The subjective sense of threat and impending danger seems to affect the lives of the inhabitants of quiet peaceful suburbs in metropolitan areas sometimes to a greater degree than communities near the border. As to the period of time since immigration to Israel, the research indicated no statistically significant difference between the participants.

The economic factor

Since 1989, parallel to immigrating to Israel, Jews left the FSU, searching for a better way of life in North American and West Europeans countries. More favourable economic conditions (the job market) also influenced a steady flow of Russian immigrants to leave Israel after a stopover of a few years, to migrate, mainly to Canada and the US: the preferred receiving emigrants' countries. This flow continues today. With few exceptions, the socio-economic position of immigrants steadily improves in their 'new' country with the passage of time; however, a gap continues to exist between the immigrants' hopes of occupational and financial success and their actual material conditions. Data also indicate that there are significant differences in nurses' salaries and work conditions between North America and Israel. Several years after immigration, social and psychological factors, such as family reunification and quality of life, rather than their material conditions, play a more important role in the well-being of immigrants (Lewin-Epstein *et al.* 2003; Lerner *et al.* 2005).

ETHICAL CONCERNS

Mireille Kingma (2001) pointed out that a delicate balance exists between human and labour rights of individual nurses and a collective concern for the health of a nation's population.

Israeli nurses strongly believe in the right to freedom of movement and choice of all individuals. We also support the ICN position statement of 2002 that stipulates nurses' right to migrate; however, it also acknowledges adverse effects of migration on the quality of healthcare in donor countries (Kline 2003). Although we have to accept the positive and negative effects of globalisation, and accept that there will always be individuals who will make their choices based on utilitarian principles, the phenomenon of unmanaged nurse migration is of growing concern. Donor countries have invested in educating nurses and do not receive a return on their investment. Does a state have the right to defend itself against the consequences?

Since healthcare organisations, private recruiters and recruitment agencies are very active internationally in recruiting foreign nurses rather than implementing changes in work conditions, we urge our policy makers, nurse managers and educators to pay more attention to the phenomenon of nurse migration, particularly with regard to the economic factor. Many nurse educators feel a sense of frustration and anger with the failure of the graduates' absorption, a real and perceived loss of valuable human resources and skilled personnel, and a loss of economic investment in education. We feel that due to the uncomplicated immigration process, many immigrants from the FSU, benefiting from Israel's resources, depart for their final destination – either to the US or Canada. We also feel impotent in the face of the extensive private recruitment efforts of these countries.

CONCLUSIONS AND RECOMMENDATIONS

The social forces directing nurse migration need to be recognised and integrated in any policy-making process addressing the issue of nurse migration. My recommendations cover three domains.

◻ **Nursing education**: The curriculum should be designed to provide a global perspective in nursing practice. More consideration should be given to developing the cultural competence of nurses. At the same time, educators and nurse managers need to examine critically the underlying organisational values of health services, such as commitment, responsibility, loyalty and devotion. Values are learned, modified and expended through education. Each student enters a nursing school with a set of values that may change during the socialisation process to reflect the values that the profession holds in high esteem. Regardless of the practice setting, professional nursing values influence the environment of nursing practice, nursing activity and the development of nursing as a profession. It is from these values that priorities will be set, standards will be developed, resources will be allocated and facets of work life will be influenced. The development of global standards of education and practice is becoming more and more important due to the increasing globalisation of professional nursing. The globalisation of education is maintained through the development of exchange programmes, international research, development of off-shore campuses and the massive increase in numbers of fee-paying overseas students (Herdman 2004). The WHO and developed as well as developing countries have begun addressing this problem in several ways, including better information and information management, effective retention studies and stronger planning processes (Oulton 2004). Developed countries are still poaching nurses from developing countries rather than improving practice conditions and education for nurses at home (Herdman 2004).

◻ **Nursing management**: Israel, like other countries at risk of nurse emigration, should adjust health sector planning. The most promising strategy for achieving international balance in the health workforce is to put more effort into building nursing resources and obtaining an adequate and sustainable source of professional nurses; i.e. by increasing the state's domestic supply of nurses. In addition, policies regarding nurse migration should be developed; these should include financial arrangements. Nursing graduates whose tuition fees were paid by the state should be required to work in the public sector for a period of time or return the money invested in their education.

☐ **Nursing research**: The growth of the migration flow, coupled with the lack of reliable data on its potential effects, should generate concerns. As of today, empirical literature regarding Israeli nurses' migration is lacking. We are unable to explain this specific phenomenon. Unfortunately, we have as yet no influence on the socio-political climate. Understanding the specific reasons for nurse migration from Israel, based on research, may help nursing managers and educators to ease the feelings of frustration, anger and sense of failure. Nurse migration is a symptom that should not be ignored.

REFERENCES

Adir Y. The Israeli Brain Drain: a psychological perspective. *Journal of Social Behavior Perspectives*. 1995; **10**(3): 731–40.

Aiken LH, Buchan J, Sochalski J, et al. Trends in International Nurse Migration. *Health Affairs*. 2004; **23**(3): 69–77.

Beenstock M, Ben-Menahem Y. The Labour Market Absorption of CIS Immigrations to Israel: 1989–1994. *International Migration*. 1997; **35**(2): 187–209.

Ben-Sira Z. *Immigration, Stress and Readjustment*. Westport, CT: Praeger; 1997.

DeAnne K, Hilfinger M. Globalization, Nursing, and Health for All. *Journal of Nursing Scholarship*. 2001; **33**(1): 9–11.

Dovlo D. Migration of Nurses from Sub-Saharan Africa: a review of issues and challenges. *Health Services Research*. 2007; **42**(3) part II: 1373–88.

Gerrish K. The Globalization of the Nursing Workforce: implication for education. *International Nurses Review*. 2004; **51**(2): 65–6.

Gould E, Moav O. *The Israeli Brain Drain*. Jerusalem: The Shalem Center, The Institute for Economic and Social Policy; 2006.

Hatton TJ, Williamson JG. *The Age of Mass Migration: causes and economic impact*. New York: Oxford University Press; 1998.

Hendel T, Fish M, Aboudi S. Strategies Used by Hospital Nurses to Cope With a National Crisis: a manager's perspective. *International Nursing Review*. 2000; **47**: 224–31.

Herdman EA. Globalization, Internationalization and Nursing. *Nursing Health Sciences*. 2004; **6**: 237–8.

Horowitz T. The Integration of Immigrants from the Former Soviet Union. *Israel Affairs*. 2005; **11**(1): 117–36.

Kaplan Z, Matar MA, Kamin R, et al. Stress-related Responses after Three Years of Exposure to Terror in Israel: are ideological-religious factors associated with resilience? *Journal of Clinical Psychiatry*. 2005; **66**: 1146–54.

Kingma M. Nursing Migration: global treasure hunt or disaster-in-the-making? *Nursing Inquiry*. 2001; **8**(4): 205–12.

Kingma M. International Perspectives. *International Nursing Review*. 2004; **51**: 196–9.

Kline DS. Push and Pull Factors in International Nurse Migration. *Journal of Nursing Scholarship*. 2003; **35**: 107–11.

Lerner Y, Kertes J, Zilber N. Immigrants from the Former Soviet Union, Five Years Post-immigration to Israel: adaptation and risk factors for psychological distress. *Psychology Medicine*. 2005; **35**: 1–10.

Lewin-Epstein N, Semyonov M, Kogan I, *et al.* Institutional Structure and Immigrant Integration: a comparative study of immigrants' labor market attainment in Canada and Israel. *International Migration Review*. 2003; **37**(2): 389–420.

Little L. Nurse Migration: a Canadian case study. *Health Service Research*. 2007; **42**(3) Part 2: 1336–53.

McElmurray BJ, Solheim K, Kishi R, *et al.* Ethical Concerns in Nursing Migration. *Journal of Professional Nursing*. 2006; **22**(4): 226–35.

Ministry of Immigration Absorption. 2007. Available at: http://www.moia.gov.il (accessed 29 January 2007).

MOH. Nursing Division Report, 2006. Available at: http://www.health.gov.il/pages/default.asp?maincat=12 (accessed 29 March 2007).

OiSaeng H. The Globalization of Occupational Health Nursing: advancing education, practice and research. *American Association of Occupational Health Nurses Journal*. 2003; **51**(2): 54.

Oulton JA. Nurse Migration: let's tackle the real issues. *International Nursing Review*. 2004; **51**: 137–8.

Ross SJ, Polsky D, Sochalski J. Nursing Shortage and International Nurse Migration. *International Nursing Review*. 2005; **52**: 253–62.

Rotem-Picker O, Toren O. Anticipated Shortage of Registered Nurses in Israel. *Achot B'yisrael* (Hebrew). 2005; **171**: 12–13.

Seloilwe ES. Globalization and Nursing. *Journal of Advanced Nursing*. 2005; **50**(6): 571.

Shalev AY, Tuval R, Frenkiel-Fishman S, *et al.* Psychological Responses to Continuous Terror: a study of two communities in Israel. *American Journal of Psychiatry*. 2006; **163**(4): 667–73.

Waters WF. Globalization, Socioeconomic Restructuring and Community Health. *Journal of Community Health*. 2001; **26**(2): 79–92.

10

Reforming (inter)national regulatory standards: the UK's failure to recognise and value the skills of overseas-trained nurses

Helen Allan

INTRODUCTION

In this chapter, I address two areas in which overseas-trained nurses' skills are not adequately recognised.

1 The failure of UK clinical managers and employers to recognise and value such nurses and their skills in the workforce.
2 The failure of the regulatory bodies to consider flexible models of assessment to determine overseas-trained nurses' skills prior to registration.

These findings are based on data from a research study that investigated overseas-trained nurses' career progression in the UK (Researching Equal Opportunities of Overseas Nurses and other Health Care Professionals (REOH). This was undertaken collaboratively by the University of Surrey, the Open University and the Royal College of Nursing (RCN) and funded by the European Social Fund.

Data from this study suggest that overseas-trained nurses' skills and competencies gained in their home countries are not recognised and valued by their employers and colleagues in the UK, and that the Nursing and Midwifery Council (NMC) has failed to provide a flexible model for assessment as proposed by Diane Wickett amd Helen McCutcheon (2002). In addition, the data suggests that, instead of being seen as trained nurses with skills to offer the workforce, they are seen as learners whose sole need is to adapt to the British nursing system. This is seen as being a one-way process of learning how the British system works rather than as a potential exchange of expertise and ideas to enhance practice. This situation is discriminatory (Henry 2007; Larsen 2006), and is shaped by empirical differences between international systems of nursing practice that lead to confusion as well as ethnocentric attitudes towards difference in the UK workforce (Allan *et al.* 2004; O'Brien 2007). It is also shaped by a discourse of 'risk' and litigation in UK health policy and practice that seeks conformity in practice. There are sponsored systems of promotion in nursing as well as markets of recruitment and employment (Allan *et al.* 2004), which mean that overseas-trained nurses are restricted in their career progression. Here I argue that overseas nurses are also systematically discriminated against because of the values underpinning accreditation; i.e. a preference for similarities in practice rather than difference.

The study

The research design allowed an in-depth understanding of overseas-trained nurses' opportunities for career development in the UK. Data collection involved individual and in-depth semi-structured interviews with overseas-trained nurses and other healthcare professionals from different backgrounds across three UK regions; interviews with national and local stakeholders and case studies involving UK healthcare employers in the National Health Service (NHS) and independent sectors in three UK regions; and case study fieldwork in one diaspora UK community and the country of origin. A total of 93 overseas healthcare professionals, 24 local and 13 national stakeholders were interviewed.

CURRENT SYSTEMS OF ACCREDITING OVERSEAS-TRAINED NURSES' QUALIFICATIONS

Wickett & McCutcheon (2002) argued that the process of assessing professional nursing qualifications globally is unnecessarily difficult and time consuming, and there are problematic issues concerning qualification assessment of nurses in a global market that have yet to be addressed by national and international bodies. They say that nurse regulatory bodies need to 'welcome diversity rather than strive for narrow uniformity' (p. 52), and that 'models for assessment need to be explored that take into account the variation in different countries' educational preparation for nurses and the range of health care settings where nurses practice' (p. 52). In addition, paper assessments where the overseas-trained nurses present their training transcript give an inadequate indication of competence in a new practice context and do not allow for recognition of experience and continuing professional development (Hancock 2002). Ailsa Masterson (2002) argues that paper assessments from overseas present particular problems: transcripts may be difficult to obtain if they were completed many years previously, they may need translation and it may be difficult to check reliability and authenticity.

Both Patricia Hancock (2002) and Masterson (2002) argue that assessment for registration in the UK of overseas-trained nurses could take place in the clinical environment. Alternatively, Masterson (2002) argues that assessment between countries could be via shared accreditation agreements outside the EU. She argues that the UK Department of Health (DH) has invested significant amounts of money to investigate overseas-trained doctors' experiences in order to produce some kind of shared accreditation, but has not investigated similar systems of accreditation for nurses or allied health professionals. Nevertheless, Masterson (2002) believes that it is unreasonable and inappropriate to expect nursing practice to be the same the world over. There are significant differences in standards of practice within and between different healthcare providers in individual countries. Masterson states that 'it might be more appropriate to ask each practitioner to prepare a portfolio of evidence against competencies expected for registration rather than evidence of registration in the qualifying country' (2002, p. 59). In addition she argues that a core competency that overseas-trained nurses need to demonstrate in their portfolio might be the ability to be flexible and transfer skills they already possess to different cultures and contexts. Even if portfolios were adopted as a system of accreditation, Masterson argues that it is difficult to estimate with any certainty how many years and how many hours per week nurses, whatever their year of training, are likely to have worked and therefore, how this experience may be expected to be recognised and valued. It is equally difficult to estimate the relationship between years of experience, educational qualifications and continuing professional education that overseas-trained nurses might reasonably expect to have assessed.

To complicate this issue further, current systems of accrediting learning in nursing, e.g. acquired prior learning (APL), acquired prior experiential learning (APEL) and acquired prior certified learning (APCL), are fairly complex, and there is no standard acceptance within the NHS about any prior training and its portability between hospitals or trusts or the independent sector (NMC 2006). Overseas-trained nurses would firstly need to show that their learning was part of their current role under the UK's Agenda for Change programme (a salary structure related to skills), and that the training is identified in their personal development plan. For example, if intravenous drug administration is part of the overseas-trained nurses' role description and they trained some time ago, they would need to demonstrate to their NHS place of employment that their past learning was compatible with what is taught now in order to be accredited. This usually involves submitting their certificate to prove they passed the course, the course programme aims and learning objectives. It is their responsibility to map these against the current training to show they have a match. They would also need to demonstrate that their level of clinical skills is up to date. Many students are required to submit a critical reflection on their clinical skills and then demonstrate them under supervision with a ward member of staff. If intravenous drug administration were not part of their role, then the employer does not have to recognise their training, although they should prepare the evidence in case they apply in the future for promotion where such skills would be required as part of the job description.

Generally APL and APCL are linked to training that carries credit for transfer (credit accumulation and transfers systems: CATS) points and are used when nurses wish to add them into an award such as a diploma or degree and, in reality, it is often easier, especially if there is a gap since nurses last practised, to retrain. NHS institutions have no obligation to honour previous continuing professional development (CPD) training. They have to recognise professional and formal academic qualifications but CPD is largely discretionary.

OVERSEAS-TRAINED NURSES' EMPLOYMENT IN THE UK

From a RCN labour force survey, Jane Ball and Geoff Pike (2005) have identified significant differences between overseas-trained nurses and UK-trained nurses (these figures are limited as they pertain only to nurses who are RCN members).

- More overseas-trained nurses are employed in independent care homes/ hospitals and bank and agency work, often in older people's nursing
- Sixty-one per cent of overseas-trained nurses are employed on D grade (newly-qualified staff nurse) compared with 14% of all UK-trained nurses. More are employed full-time, despite the fact that equal numbers have dependent children
- More overseas-trained nurses work shifts on an internal rotation format; 44% work 11-hour shifts compared with 27% of UK-trained nurses
- Fewer overseas-trained nurses have a nursing diploma but a larger number have a degree.

The following tables show that the overseas-trained nurses interviewed for the REOH study were more likely to be employed in the NHS compared with those in the RCN survey (Ball & Pike 2005). There are also other differences. The following data show the date the nurses arrived in the UK, their current employer, current grade, ethnicity by grade, year of registration in the home country and qualifications overseas.

In Table 10.1, it can be seen that 20% of the nurses sampled arrived before 2000, with the majority of overseas-trained nurses arriving after that date.

TABLE 10.1 Date of arrival in UK

1968–69	2 (2%)
1970–79	4 (4%)
1980–89	6 (6%)
1990–99	7 (8%)
2000	8 (9%)
2001	15 (16%)
2002	17 (18%)
2003	14 (15%)
2004	8 (9%)
Born in UK	1 (1%)
Unknown/not listed	11 (12%)

Table 10.2 shows that the majority of our sample was employed in the NHS rather than in independent care homes/hospitals, bank or agency work as reported by Ball and Pike (2005).

TABLE 10.2 Current employer

NHS	59 (63%)
Care/nursing home	13 (14%)
Independent	11 (12%)
Ghana Health Service	6 (6%)
Student in Ghana	2 (2%)
NHS/Private	1 (1%)
Unknown	2 (2%)

Across all sectors, nurses in our survey were employed as D grades, with a small minority of older Ghanaians employed as F or G grades (Figure 10.1). Given Ball and Pike's (2005) finding that 61% of overseas-trained nurses (RCN members) are employed as D grades in the independent and care-home sector, the majority of our sample working mainly in the NHS and arriving after 1999 also appear to be employed as D grades. There is a slight tendency for white overseas-trained nurses to be employed on higher grades.

The majority of the nurses interviewed for our survey were registered in their home country before 2000, with the largest proportion registering between 1990 and 1999; 46% were registered before 1990 (Table 10.3).

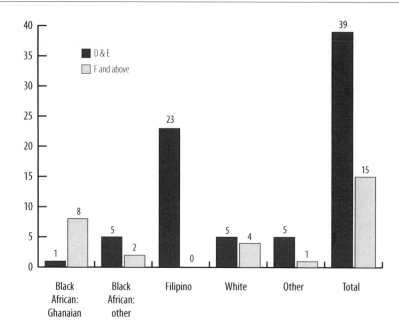

FIGURE 10.1 Ethnicity by grade

TABLE 10.3 Year of registration in home country

1968–69	1
1970–79	11
1980–89	22
1990–99	32
2000	1
Unknown/not listed	26

Given their experience, the nurses in our survey had a range of post-registration experiences and continuing professional development, as well as academic qualifications, that are currently not recognised or accredited routinely by their employers if one takes grade as an indicator. For example, 21% of the nurses in our study had dual registration in their home country, with 10 overseas-trained nurses registered as midwives in their home country; none were registered as midwives in the UK, whereas the three overseas-trained registered mental health nurses (RMNs) were also RMNs in the UK. Thirty per cent of the sample had a BSc or MSc (Table 10.4).

TABLE 10.4 Professional qualifications gained overseas

Registered nurse (RN) community, psychiatric	1 (1%)
RN midwifery BSc, MSc	1 (1%)
RN	20 (22%)
RN BSc	25 (27%)
RN BSc, MSc	2 (2%)
RN RM (Registered midwife)	9 (10%)
RN RMN	3 (3%)
Unknown/not listed	18 (19%)

It is clear from these data that the overseas-trained nurses interviewed in our study were experienced nurses before migrating to work in the UK. As with the RCN study *We Need Respect* (Allan *et al.* 2003), one would expect that these overseas-trained nurses' qualifications and experiences are enough to qualify them for senior grades, given that the majority were also working full-time, and full-time working is associated with higher grades in nursing. Instead, the majority were employed as D grades.

BEING SEEN AS LEARNERS AND NOT AS TRAINED NURSES

Empirical differences in training are expected by overseas-trained nurses who are aware that their training has been different from that in the UK. Indeed, with some variation between nationalities and social backgrounds, overseas-trained nurses' discussion of professional development revealed that learning from their British experience was one motivation for migrating to the UK. Nurses from the Indian subcontinent talked at greater length and in more detail than the other groups about training and education as their primary motivation for migration. In addition to better salaries in the UK, many African nurses, particularly from Nigeria and, to a lesser extent, South Africa, emphasised developing their skills, knowledge and careers through access to resources that would enable them to be more effective nurses. There was an expectation that they would need 'local' adaptation, but that they would be treated as trained nurses. Therefore, the period of supervised practice during their adaptation required to obtain their personal identification number (PIN) from the NMC was a source of considerable discontent, because they felt they were not respected as trained nurses, but treated as learners with no experience (Smith *et al.* 2006). There was confusion over the accreditation of their training, and a surprise that their skills gained overseas were not recognised. A Zimbabwean nurse said:

I thought I would work as soon as I came here. I thought the adaptation was just a formality. I thought I'd be accepted onto the UK register and then I would be working in a place where I would be accepted because of my experience. And then I would be working because of my experience. I thought I'd go straight into a higher grade.

This situation led to feelings of frustration as three Filipino nurses discussed during their interview:

Nurse 1:   You can't catheterise without the course.
Researcher: Even female patients?
Nurse 2:   Yes. Because previously, if you're intensive care [trained], you're equipped to do all these things because you're in critical. But if nobody's around, nobody's around to help you in case of emergency. So we are all trained there back home, but because we are legally not allowed to do so, you expected to do things that you are doing before and you can't do now.
Nurse 3:   You can't do now, because you'll go insane.
Researcher: How did that make you feel?
Nurse 1:   Frustration. Because your skills will be gone if we're not doing it. This is where I started before.

Our data suggest that UK healthcare employers, both in the care homes and the NHS, are not sufficiently prepared to meet the different learning needs of overseas-trained nurses. Generally, there was a lack of organisational thinking around how cultural differences in training and nursing practice affect mentoring and learning for both overseas-trained nurses and their mentors. No one we interviewed had considered that overseas-trained nurses might have different learning styles and learning needs compared with British nurses. As a result, overseas-trained nurses did not have their needs as trained nurses met in mentoring systems, and were treated the same as newly qualified nurses, as the following comment shows:

We basically treat them as newly-qualified members of staff with no experience until we find out what their experience is.

The focus of their adaptation period appeared to be on their learning rather than on their practical competencies. In the following quote from a mentor about an overseas-trained nurse, she comments on the nurse's learning style, the failure to produce the 'work' rather than her practical skills:

I find students challenging who just don't have the . . . they need to push. At the moment, we don't know how hard we have to push them in terms of producing the work. We're doing all the teaching, but she's not producing the work. I said to her, 'This is the beginning; you're a month and a half into it. You've got six months to do it. If you don't get this work done, it's going to be so backlogged that you won't get through.' She still hasn't produced the written work. When we're doing assistance and teaching her, she's managing to do it. It's just that she's not giving us the work so we can say yes she can do it. I said to her, 'If we don't sign you off, you can't do it.'

In response to a question about the integration of overseas standards and practices into British nursing practice, the following reply was given by a spokesperson from the NMC:

What we're saying is that these are people who are nurses, they have a lot of skills. The competency part is about confirming that they conform to our standards. We don't want a queue of people from outside coming to complain about standards and failure to protect the public. But we recognise that many of these applicants are skilled and can make a positive contribution to the service. We're delighted to welcome them if they conform to our requirements.

It was also clear from the managers' interviews that very little thought had been given to overseas-trained nurses' promotion based on their extensive skills and experience gained overseas:

Researcher: I just wondered whether you can see them being employed immediately on an E grade? Would any of them have the experience?

Manager: That's an interesting question. I'll be honest with you. I haven't even thought of that one . . . I think the issue of the grade, I hadn't considered that.

Treating overseas-trained as newly qualified nurses through lack of recognition of previous experience (APL, APEL, APCL as well as CPD) led to de-skilling (Filipino nurses), and arises because of the nature of British nursing work and the avoidance of risk. I have argued (Allan 2007) that the legal framework within which UK nurses work, which has arisen because of the delegation of medical tasks to nurses at the same time as the emergence of a discourse of 'risk' and litigation (Richman & Mercer 2004; Watson 2001), was different from their experiences in their home countries or overseas and made the experience of adaptation to British nursing more challenging. However, de-skilling also arises because of an expectation that overseas-trained nurses will adopt British nursing practices and as a result, their skills or ways of practice learnt overseas, which are different from British practices, are ignored by their British mentors and co-workers.

Overseas-trained nurses recognised that their previous experience and skills were not the reason for being recruited and, therefore, passed themselves off as less experienced or as more junior members of staff to fit into the UK nurses' expectations of overseas-trained nurses. As one Filipino overseas-trained nurse said about her previous experience and qualifications as an instructor:

> Researcher: Why don't you tell them?
> Nurse: I'm embarrassed about it. In my CV I put staff nurse as they
>   required a staff nurse. They need the staff nurse, so you had to
>   show them you were a better staff nurse. Most of my time at work
>   had been as a clinical instructor. No managerial.
> Researcher: So you had to present a different profile here?
> Nurse: Yes. That's why I didn't tell them.
> Researcher: When you go for an E grade would you tell them?
> Nurse: Yes. It's not fair but there is a difficulty for British nurses having
>   more qualified overseas nurses working with them.

This approach among British nurses to ignore non-UK experience and skills gained overseas led some overseas-trained nurses to downgrade their experiences and skills so as not to appear arrogant, and to allow them to get on better with UK colleagues, who placed overseas-trained nurses at the bottom of ward hierarchy and did not expect much from them. As this Filipino nurse said:

> Researcher: Do you think they realise how much experience you have?
> Nurse: They do, maybe that's why they don't like us and avoid us. When
>   I was in ICU they told me 'Oh, you're a senior nurse'. I was very
>   careful in my work, like every time I do things I was very careful.
>   They might look and say something bad. They might criticise.
>   I have to be careful; not perfect, but I've learnt to be humble for
>   them. It's like they are the superiors. I cannot act like a superior.

DISCUSSION

Fluctuating nurse recruitment has been a feature of British nursing since 1948, and recruitment of overseas-trained and untrained staff has been a response to recruitment crises since then. Our data suggest that overseas-trained nurses are recruited primarily to fulfil the workforce demands of the NHS at D-grade level rather than to contribute to workforce development at higher grades (Hardill & MacDonald 2000; Smith *et al.* 2006). This situation is also happening in Australia (Hawthorne 2001; Konno 2006). The lack of flexibility in mentoring systems, and the lack of thinking about the potential contribution of overseas-trained nurses to workforce development may arise from viewing overseas-trained nurses simply as learners instead of seeing them as trained nurses with skills to offer the workforce.

There is a need to develop a more flexible approach to recognising and valuing overseas-trained nurses' skills for several reasons. Firstly, there is the increasing globalisation of nursing and movement of nurses internationally (Kingma 2003; Winkelmann-Gleed 2005). It is only recently that the UK government has finally acknowledged the legacy of international recruitment from the Caribbean in the 1950s and 1960s, and addressed inequalities in its black and minority ethnic workforce (Smith *et al.* 2006). Therefore, lessons must be learnt now from what is an established pattern of the global migration of nurses to make the experiences of overseas-trained nurses better. Secondly, by viewing overseas-trained nurses as unskilled, the NHS is not making the most of resources and talents in the migrant workforce. Thirdly, the delivery of high-quality patient care can be improved by utilising highly skilled overseas-trained nurses. Lastly, the important risk-management issues can be addressed flexibly through portfolio evidence of previous experience overseas and single assessment of a particular skill and competency or a period of supervised practice of a skill to ensure that local safety standards are met. These benefits to the NHS can be realised only if overseas-trained nurses are supported and valued as members of the workforce (Gerrish & Griffith 2004; Smith *et al.* 2006).

CONCLUSIONS

I have illustrated, with some empirical data from the experiences of overseas-trained nurses, how British employers and clinical managers have dealt with the increasing globalisation of the nursing workforce to date. NHS managers and employers interviewed have not even begun to think about how they might value difference and utilise overseas-trained nurses' experiences and skills meaningfully in the NHS workforce. This is in part due to poor leadership from the NMC and the DH, who have not led thinking around how developing systems of assessing overseas-trained nurses' qualifications and experiences might be developed. Either the regulatory authorities, the DH, or NHS employers and clinical managers need to address these issues in order to captialise on the rich and diverse experiences brought to the NHS by overseas-trained nurses. The workforce issues emerging from an international and transitory health and social care workforce need to be addressed nationally and globally with leadership from international and national regulatory bodies. Failure to do so will increase overseas-trained nurses' experiences of isolation and alienation.

REFERENCES

Allan HT. The Rhetoric of Caring and the Recruitment of Overseas Nurses: the social production of a care gap. *Journal of Clinical Nursing Special Issue.* 2007; **16**: 2204–12.

Allan HT, Larsen JA. *We Need Respect: experiences of internationally recruited nurses in the* UK. Report to the Royal College of Nursing. 2003. Available at: http://www.rcn.org.uk/__data/assets/pdf_file/0008/78587/002061.pdf (accessed 5 May 2008).

Allan HT, Larsen JA, Bryan K, Smith PA. The Social Reproduction of Institutional Racism: internationally recruited nurses' experiences of the British Health Services. *Diversity in Health and Social Care.* 2004; **1**(2): 117–26.

Ball J, Pike G. *Managing to Work Differently: results from the* RCN *employment survey 2005.* London: RCN; 2005.

Gerrish K, Griffith V. Integration of Overseas Registered Nurses: evaluation of an adaptation programme. *Journal of Advanced Nursing.* 2004; **45**(6): 579–87.

Hancock PK. Commentary: a response to Diane Wickett and Helen McCutcheon. Issues of qualification assessment for nurses in a global market (*Nurse Education Today.* 2002; **22**(1): 44–52). Nurse Education Today. 2002; **22**(1): 53–56.

Hardill I, MacDonald S. Skilled International Migration: the experience of nursing in the UK. *Regional Studies.* 2000; **34**(7): 681–92.

Hawthorne K. The globalisation of the nursing workforce: barriers confronting overseas qualified nurses in Australia. *Nursing Inquiry.* 2001; **8**(4): 213–29.

Henry L. Institutionalized Disadvantage: older Ghanaian nurses' and midwives' reflections on career progression and stagnation in the NHS. *Journal of Clinical Nursing.* 2007; **16**: 2196–203.

Kingma M. *Nurses on the Move: migration and the global health care economy.* Ithaca, NY: Cornell University Press; 2003.

Konno R. Support for Overseas Qualified Nurses in Adjusting to Australian Nursing Practice: a systematic review. *International Journal of Evidence-based Healthcare.* 2006; **4**(2): 83–100.

Larsen JA. *Fitting in and moving on: cultural habituation and career progression for overseas nurses.* Paper presented at the Royal College of Nursing International Research Conference, York, UK: 21–24 March 2006.

Masterson A. Commentary: a response to Diane Wickett and Helen McCutcheon. Issues of qualification assessment for nurses in a global market (*Nurse Education Today.* 2002; 22(1): 44–52). Nurse Education Today. 2002; **22**(1): 57–59.

NMC. *A–Z Advice Sheet Accreditation of prior and experiential learning (APEL) and credit accumulation transfer schemes (CATS).* 2006. Available at: www.nmc-uk.org (accessed 30 July 2007).

O'Brien T. Overseas Nurses (OSN) in the National Health Service (NHS): a process of deskilling. *Journal of Clinical Nursing Special Issue.* 2007; **16**(12): 2229–36.

Richman R, Mercer D. Modern Language or Spin: nursing newspeak and organisational culture: new health scriptures. *Journal of Nursing Management.* 2004; **12**(5): 290–8.

Smith PA, Allan HT, Henry L, *et al. Valuing and Recognising the Talents of a Diverse Healthcare Workforce.* Report to the European Social Fund on Researching Equal Opportunities of Overseas Nurses and other Health Care Professionals. 2006. Available at: http//:portal.surrey.ac.uk/reoh (accessed 29 March 2008).

Watson R. Friends in low places. *Journal of Advanced Nursing.* 2001; **236**(2): 321.

Wickett D, McCutcheon H. Issues of Qualification Assessment for Nurses in a Global Market. *Nurse Education Today.* 2002; **22**(1): 44–52.

Winkelmann-Gleed A. *Migrant Nurses Motivation, Integration and Contribution.* London: Routledge; 2005.

11

Disengagement and demoralisation: the roots of Ghanaian nurses' responses to discrimination in the (UK) NHS

Leroi Henry

INTRODUCTION

Since 1999, nurses trained overseas have made up almost half of new entrants to the profession as recorded on the Nursing and Midwifery Council (NMC) register (NMC 2004; NMC 2007). This reflects a pattern established in the middle of the last century whereby the UK healthcare system has periodically suffered acute labour shortages that have been resolved by recruiting migrants, primarily from the Commonwealth and Ireland (Smith & Macintosh 2007). The most recent wave of migration has provoked much discussion worldwide about the ethics of the globalisation of healthcare labour markets. While the general characteristics of migrant nurses have been mapped (Buchan & Dovlo 2004; Buchan *et al.* 2005), with some notable exceptions (Allan & Larson 2003; Allan *et al.* 2004), there has been relatively little detailed research on migrant nurses' experiences in the increasingly globalised labour market. This chapter focuses on how nurses perceived discriminatory practices and structures, how they responded to them, and how these can have both positive and negative outcomes when resisting or entrenching discrimination. This is based on data collected by the author and other researchers as part of the REOH project (*see* Chapter 10), a research study that investigated overseas-trained nurses' career progression in the UK. This was undertaken collaboratively by the Open University, the University of Surrey and the Royal College of Nursing and was financed by the European Social Fund.

The chapter builds on previous REOH work on discriminatory practices and structures in career progression in the UK NHS, with particular reference to promotion into management (Henry 2007; Smith *et al.* 2006). It explores Ghanaian nurses' and midwives' responses to these practices, and discusses how some responses to perceived racism entrench the marginalisation and exclusion of those affected. The emphasis is on the importance of individual agency in determining the outcomes of discrimination by exploring how responses to structural racism and discriminatory practices relate to migration strategies and, in turn, impact on career progression.

METHODOLOGY

The data were gathered through semi-structured interviews with 20 nurses and midwives trained in Ghana and currently working in the UK. This group constituted an embedded case study (Yin 1994) within a larger sample of over 100 informants of different nationalities. Informants were located through a combination of networking and snowballing strategies, including:

☐ utilising contacts from previous research (Henry & Mohan 2003; Allan & Larson 2003)
☐ accessing diaspora communities through addressing meetings of associations
☐ case study visits at healthcare workplaces in the NHS and independent healthcare providers in London and the Home Counties (i.e. the counties around London); these case studies involved interviews with overseas-trained nurses and local stakeholders, including clinical and senior managers
☐ snowballing from the above contacts.

The informants were mostly well established in the UK, had a great deal of experience and had adapted to working in the NHS with varying degrees of success. They were mostly F- and G-grade nurses and midwives (see Appendix, pp. 124–5), with over half being in the UK for over 15 years. The data were supplemented by three more recent migrants working on lower grades. All interviewees were working full-time in NHS hospitals in London and the Home Counties. Almost all had UK or dual nationality, and had their families in the UK. The sample is not intended to be representative of Ghanaian nurses and midwives in the UK, as recent migrants on lower grades and healthcare assistants are under-represented.

Interviews were undertaken either in participants' homes or at a local branch of the Open University. Interviews were semi-structured using an interview guide and were audio-recorded; the aims of the project were explained; anonymity was guaranteed, and interviewees read and signed a consent form. The interview guide was structured around four sections: personal details, key events and equal opportunities, key themes and social networks. The first section provided general personal and current employment data. The second explored such key events as securing the participant's current post and first post in the UK, promotion and training. The issues raised in this section were discussed in more detail in the third section focusing on working conditions, relationships with colleagues, patients and managers, and adapting to the UK. The fourth section explored the role of social networks and support systems.

The interviews lasted around one-and-a-half hours. The audio-recordings were transcribed verbatim and then coded using data analysis software (NVivo, version 2.0). All REOH researchers used a common set of codes to facilitate cross-case analysis. Each interview was given attributes detailing key variables to facilitate cross-case data retrieval. The first five interviews by each researcher were verified by the research team and the coding strategy was updated after reaching consensus. The research team held regular meetings over the period of the project to develop and confirm one another's empirical findings and theoretical insights as the research progressed.

Research in the UK was supplemented by field work in Ghana, which I undertook with a Ghanaian researcher. This involved semi-structured interviews and focus groups with about 40 doctors, nurses and final-year medical and nursing students at the two largest hospitals and at a smaller rural hospital. The purpose of this fieldwork was to cross-check discourses on the career structure and organisational culture in the Ghanaian healthcare system, and to provide a reference point to research on migrants' aspirations and discourses of success and failure.

MIGRATION MOTIVATIONS

In order to understand how migrant nurses and midwives conceptualise their experiences in the workplace, one must first contextualise them in relation to their reasons for migration. Given the increasingly integrated international nursing labour market (Mensah *et al.* 2005; Mackintosh *et al.* 2006), the salary differentials between nurses in high-income and low-income countries are often perceived to be the sole explanatory factor for nurse migration. However, there is significant evidence that the process is more complex (Vujicic *et al.* 2004, Smith *et al.* 2006). For the informants, the primary motivation for migration to the UK was material advancement. For them, *doing* nursing in the UK was a means to achieve material ends as opposed to *being* a nurse in the UK as an end in itself. This is related to a desire for increased remuneration and improved quality of life for themselves and their immediate families. While they also had obligations to their parental household and other members of the extended family, meeting these obligations was not stated as a primary reason for migration.

Their notions of material advancement were strongly transnational as, in addition to supporting relatives, all the informants were engaged in developing assets back in Ghana. In particular, all but one of the informants were building houses in Accra and/or the ancestral hometown; a smaller number had invested in business opportunities in Ghana. Their long-term investments were a response to inadequate remuneration for healthcare professionals and also to the lack of access to credit in Ghana. The extent and nature of their investments reflected the fact that most wanted to work in the UK for an extended period of time but intended to return to Ghana. This was reflected in the immigration status of the participants, as all but one had dual Ghanaian and UK citizenship.

CAREER PROGRESSION IN THE NHS

There are limited statistical data available on the career progression of overseas-trained nurses; however some trends can be discerned from the RCN labour force survey (Ball & Pike 2005). According to this survey, in comparison with their UK-trained counterparts, overseas-trained nurses are overwhelmingly concentrated in lower grades, with 61% of overseas-trained nurses employed on D grade (newly-qualified staff nurse level) compared with 14% of all UK-trained nurses (Ball & Pike 2005). It should be noted that these statistics refer only to RCN members who responded to the survey, and do not differentiate between different groups of overseas-trained nurses (*see* also Chapter 10).

Previous research by REOH has considered these statistics by exploring nurses' perceptions of inappropriate grading and under-utilisation of skills, and the difficulties they have experienced in promotion into managerial posts (Henry 2007; Smith *et al.* 2006).

Many of the informants experienced difficulties in adapting to career advancement in the NHS, which they initially tended to attribute to socio-cultural differences, and particularly to communication skills rather than clinical skills. Many experienced difficulties in performing well in interviews, and found it difficult to use buzzwords and professional discourses to demonstrate their nursing skills. However, their disadvantage was entrenched and institutionalised by a lack of support from managers in addressing their specific needs as overseas-trained staff. Most informants had experienced practices and structures, including access to training, quality of training, and opportunities to gain experience of management through 'acting up', i.e. deputising for a senior person, they labelled as discriminatory on the basis of race or ethnicity. Many participants alleged discrimination in the quality of support given to them in the promotion process, particularly in interview preparation and feedback. They believed that chosen candidates were pre-selected and coached while others were ignored or received inadequate or misleading support. Promotion into management resembled systems of patronage based on meeting subjective and culturally specific criteria that provided a space for racial and ethnic discrimination (Henry 2007).

STAGNATION, ALIENATION, DEMORALISATION AND DISENGAGEMENT

For many nurses and midwives, the result of discrimination meant career stagnation. They remained on the same grade for years, despite regularly applying for promotion, but consistently failing without being given adequate explanation and without receiving any meaningful support from their clinical managers. One midwife outlined her frustrations:

> While I was (acting up) I went for an interview for the proper job. I didn't get it. The following year I went; I didn't get it. The following year I went; I didn't get it. And then the fourth time I was doing this – I was in charge of the unit department – and I went the fourth time and I didn't get it. So I got frozen . . . I felt that I wasn't getting any help. I was working but I wasn't getting any help. I got so frustrated . . . I'm so hurt and it's so painful you know, I'm grieving. It's like I'm good, I'm doing my work well, but it seems I'm marching but I'm not moving forward.

Many of the Ghanaian nurses and midwives perceived that managers favoured white or African Caribbean nurses over Africans and that, consequently, these ethnic groups are promoted far more quickly. They believed that their long periods of career stagnation and under-achievement were caused by endemic racial or ethnic discrimination, and reinforced by a perception of a lack of support or interest from managers. As a reaction to repeated failure to progress, many more participants than can be quoted became alienated from their workplace and managers, and many became deeply demoralised. To shield themselves from what they saw as a humiliating process, they disengaged from career progression and adopted what appears to be an increasingly instrumental attitude to their professional life by focusing on their job as a means to an end rather than gaining intrinsic satisfaction from it. This is evident in the following comment from a F-grade midwife:

> I'm really fed up and I just don't want to know anymore. I think I will just be where I am, just get my money to pay the mortgage and that's the attitude, which is bad but at the end of the day, I don't know; probably I feel I can't get anywhere anymore. There was a time I just felt so de-motivated I just couldn't be bothered, honestly. I just didn't even want to go on any course or anything because I felt I can't get any further so why should I bother.

Another nurse stated:

I don't think my face fits so I won't even bother because, when you go for interviews and you don't get it, it's really depressing; it demoralises you and me, in particular, it takes months to overcome it.

In this process of demoralisation and alienation, the traumas and frustrations engendered by past and ongoing discrimination have become internalised by the victims, who now seek to avoid exposing themselves to further humiliation.

The disengagement from career progression and career development included ceasing to apply for jobs and promotion, not updating skills and avoiding responsibility. This seems to be widespread and widely acknowledged by Ghanaian nurses. However, some nurses had developed strategies to resist discrimination and had been more successful in gaining promotion. While some of this group had given support and advice to others, many often continued to experience demoralisation. A Ghanaian midwifery manager stated:

You just had to work harder, have more qualifications, do more and at the end of the day you think, 'Is it really worth it?' It's not really worth it for the stress. You might as well earn your money and go home. For me, to go any further along, I just can't be bothered. I'm just going to enjoy life. It's not worth it.

SUCCESSFUL MIGRATION AND RESISTING VICTIMHOOD

These responses of alienation from the workplace and withdrawal from career progression must be understood in the context of the migrants' original aims, and how these aims change in relation to labour market needs and changing personal circumstances. The definitions of successful migration used by informants focus on material advancement and improved quality of life for themselves and their immediate families rather than on career advancement. Hence many stressed that, once established in the UK, the most important issue for the nurses and midwives who have children in Ghana was to be in a financial and legal position to bring them over from Ghana. This then led to the need to balance their careers with other commitments and interests, as their choices of career direction were constrained by their responsibilities. Almost all the participants also had strong obligations to relatives in Ghana; however, they claimed that these obligations had no impact on their career strategies. While these obligations did not determine the direction of migrants' careers, having the capacity to support the extended family financially was deemed as a critical indicator of status as a migrant.

Many of the nurses who have not been successful in gaining promotion have instead focused on other aspects of their lives, such as their immediate family in the UK or their extended family, property and investments in Ghana. Most of the informants originally aimed to move between the UK and Ghanaian nursing labour market. None of the UK-based sample had been able to circulate in this way owing to UK immigration controls, family commitments and a strong perception that the UK experience is not valued by the Ghanaian Health Service. However, most were planning for their retirement or return to Ghana to work in the private sector. This reflects the dual identity that most Ghanaian migrants maintained, expressed as 'living both here and there' (Henry & Mohan 2003). All the healthcare professionals owned land or property (houses, businesses) in Ghana. This emphasis on people and places in Ghana can be seen as re-orienting themselves to the original reasons for migrating to the UK, remuneration and material advancement for themselves and their immediate families rather than for the professional space to develop their careers (Smith *et al.* 2006). This is evident in the comments of a midwife, who illustrates that career stagnation does not necessarily equate to failure as a migrant.

> I was just hoping to get a higher grade, get more money and then just go home, have my clinic and help my people back home . . . but now I don't think I will bother about the G grade. My salary is a little bit increased now with the new pay structure, so what I do is just a bit of agency work to top it up if I need something extra.

BECOMING AN AGENT IN ONE'S OWN MARGINALISATION

The participants' responses to perceived institutional and direct discrimination involve a process of alienation from the workplace and disengagement from career progression. They do not imply that migrants have failed to achieve their own objectives. However, the effects of discrimination led to a lack of career progression, with the nurses and midwives having effectively become agents in their own marginalisation. The widespread alienation and disengagement from careers reflects a hidden but potentially pervasive dimension of the disadvantage of the marginalised position of many black and minority ethnic (particularly African) staff in the NHS. In response to a history of perceived discrimination, the victims themselves add a further dimension of racism.

This dimension can be understood as black and minority ethnic and/or overseas nurses not being interested in or not capable of career progression. Withdrawal from career progression can become an explanation in itself, rather than be a starting point for examining processes and structures in the NHS to explain why disengagement from career progression is so common in some groups of overseas-trained staff. If managers perceive that it is not their responsibility to address discriminatory practices, processes or institutional barriers because the practitioners themselves render them irrelevant by their own actions, then in the context of limited support in the workplace, it is easier for managers to do nothing. A cycle of denial of underlying problems related to clinical performance or interpersonal skills is then maintained, leading to further disengagement and dissatisfaction

The process of marginalisation can become self-sustaining as it feeds back into further alienation and demoralisation. A history of perceived racism led the group of African nurses and midwives who participated in this study to expect to meet racism, become alienated and demoralised, therefore as a group and as individuals their responses to marginalisation became entrenched and self-fulfilling.

Focusing on the negative effects of responses to perceived discrimination is in no way blaming these professionals for their predicament. It is an understandable response that is closely related to their original aims as migrants and is also possibly a reflection on the age and family obligations of the informants, and is gender-related. It does not deny the context of structural discrimination in the NHS and discriminatory practices that have provoked these responses in the first place. The purpose of this analysis is to understand how and why people have responded to discrimination in different ways and to highlight the effects of these adaptations on their careers. Highlighting the importance of reactions to discrimination broadens our conceptual focus beyond discriminatory structures and practices to include the impact of collective and individual agency on the outcomes for individuals and groups.

CONCLUSIONS

Ghanaian-trained nurses and midwives who work in the NHS perceived discrimination in career progression, leading to alienation, demoralisation and disengagement. This led to marginalisation of this group, feeding into a self-sustaining and self-fulfilling narrative of discrimination that became a lens through which negative experiences in the workplace were interpreted. It must be remembered, though, that the sample size and type makes it difficult to generalise from these data. More research is needed on this topic.

REFERENCES

Allan HT, Larsen JA. We Need Respect: experiences of internationally recruited nurses in the UK. Report to the Royal College of Nursing. 2003. Available at: http://www.rcn.org.uk/__data/assets/pdf_file/0008/78587/002061.pdf (accessed 5 May 2008).

Allan HT, Larsen JA, Bryan K, Smith P. The Social Reproduction of Institutional Racism: internationally recruited nurses' experiences of the British health services. Diversity in Health and Social Care. 2004; 1(2): 117–26.

Ball J, Pike G. *Managing to Work Differently: results from the RCN employment survey 2005*. London: RCN; 2005. Available at http://www.rcn.org.uk/publications/pdf/aes_2005.pdf (accessed 30 September 2007).

Buchan J, Dovlo, D. *International Recruitment of Health Workers to the UK: a report for the Department for International Development*. 2004. Available at http://www.dfidhealthrc.org/publications/country_information/int-rec-main.pdf (accessed 30 September 2007).

Buchan J, Gough P, Hutt R. *Internationally Recruited Nurses in London: profile and implications for policy*. London: King's Fund; 2005.

Henry L. Institutionalized Disadvantage: older Ghanaian nurses' and midwives' reflections on career progression and stagnation in the NHS. *Journal of Clinical Nursing*. 2007; **16**: 2196–203.

Henry L, Mohan G. Making Homes: the Ghanaian diaspora, institutions and development. *Journal of International Development*. 2003; **15**: 611–22.

Mackintosh M, Mensah K, Henry L, Rowson M. Aid, Restitution and International Fiscal Redistribution in Health Care: implications of health professionals' migration. *Journal of International Development*. 2006; **18**: 757–70.

Mensah K, Mackintosh M, Henry L. *The Skills Drain of Health Professionals in the Developing World*. London: Medact; 2005. Available at: http://www.medact.org/content/Skills%20drain/Mensah%20et%20al.%202005.pdf (accessed 30 September 2007).

NMC. *Statistical Analysis of the Register 1 April 2003 to 31 March 2004*. London: NMC; 2004. Available at: http://www.nmc-uk.org/aFrameDisplay.aspx?DocumentID=602 (accessed 30 September 2007).

NMC. *Statistical Analysis of the Register 1 April 2005 to 31 March 2006*. London: NMC; 2007. Available at: http://www.nmc-uk.org/aFrameDisplay.aspx?DocumentID=2593 (accessed 30 September 2007).

Smith PA, Allan HT, Henry L, *et al*. *Valuing and Recognising the Talents of a Diverse Healthcare Workforce*. Report to the European Social Fund on Researching Equal Opportunities of Overseas Nurses and other Health Care Professionals. 2006. Available at: http://portal.surrey.ac.uk/pls/portal/docs/PAGE/REOH/LAU/REOH%20REPORT%20070706.PDF (accessed 30 September 2007).

Smith P, Mackintosh M. Profession, Market and Class: nurse migration and the remaking of hierarchy and disadvantage. *Journal of Clinical Nursing Special Issue*. 2007; **16**: 2213–20.

Vujicic M, Zurn P, Daillo K, *et al*. The Role of Wages in the Migration of Health Care Professionals From Developing Countries. *Human Resources for Health*. 2004; **2**: 3.

Yin R. *Case Study Research: design and methods*. London: Sage; 1994.

APPENDIX: CAREER GRADE STRUCTURE IN THE UK

A first-year nursing student

B second-year nursing student

C third-year nursing student

D Newly-qualified junior staff nurse

E Staff nurse

F Senior staff nurse, junior charge nurse or team leader

G Sister, charge nurse or ward manager

H Nursing manager responsible for several wards or departments, or clinical specialist

I Senior nursing manager

SECTION 4

Religion and ethnicity

12

Nursing, Islamic fundamentalism and terrorism

Leyla Dinç and Verena Tschudin

INTRODUCTION

In the non-Islamic world, Islam is often portrayed as an enigmatic entity. Much of what is seen and heard about Islam is associated with unrest, terrorism and fear. This makes it inevitable that nurses meet this aspect, too, when caring for patients from Muslim countries or those who may have been affected by recent wars and terror attacks. It is important that nurses have an understanding of the roots of terrorism and fundamentalism, especially as they apply to Islam. However, they need to be seen in a wider political and social context, and nurses are in prime positions to explain the threat, causes and consequences of terrorism and help to prevent it.

In 1948, the UN recognised the importance of freedom of religion in the Universal Declaration of Human Rights (UN 1948). Article 18 states that:

> Everyone has the right to freedom of thought, conscience and religion; this right includes freedom to change his religion or belief, and freedom, either alone or in community with others and in public or private, to manifest his religion or belief in teaching, practice, worship and observance.

Article 30 states:

> Nothing in this Declaration may be interpreted as implying for any State, group or person any right to engage in any activity or to perform any act aimed at the destruction of any of the rights and freedoms set forth herein.

In this context, respect for human rights encompasses a notion that includes religious freedom as long as it does not infringe on the rights and freedoms of others.

The ICN *Code of Ethics for nurses* (ICN 2006) makes it clear that nurses have a fundamental responsibility to respect human rights and to provide care that is unrestricted by considerations of age, colour, creed, culture, religion, disability or illness, gender, nationality, politics, race or social status. It also stipulates four fundamental responsibilities that nurses have: 'to promote health, to prevent illness, to restore health and to alleviate suffering'. These responsibilities have to be seen in the context of issues that influence the health of all people, such as poverty, unemployment, global inequalities, wars and terrorism. There are 11 million nurses working around the world and nurses are the largest group of health professionals. The collective voice of such a power base can have a large impact in favour of global justice and a peaceful future, especially for the prevention of terrorism. In order to do this, nurses have to have an understanding of the issues involved. This chapter outlines these in general, and in particular in relation to Islam.

The attacks on the World Trade Center in New York on 11 September 2001, and subsequent attacks such as those in Istanbul, Madrid and London, perpetuated by terrorists in the name of Islam, caused thousands of deaths. The attacks demonstrated that terrorism can cross borders and can affect anyone or any place at any time. The health consequences of these attacks were enormous and disastrous. Survivors suffered from various injuries and mental health problems, including depression, anxiety and post-traumatic stress disorder (Miguel-Tobal *et al.* 2006; Moline *et al.* 2006). In the aftermath of the September 11 attack, a large number of people sustained potential exposure to smoke, dust, and a variety of toxins, which increases the risk of respiratory diseases and cancer (Moline *et al.* 2006). Nurses were the first responders and they played an important role in caring for victims and survivors. These unexpected attacks indicated that nurses need to be aware and prepared for the health consequences of terrorism (Silva & Ludwick 2003).

The ICN published resources for coping with terrorism, including information, ethical guidelines, position statements and links to provide nurses with tools to assist in coping and caring for victims of terrorist attacks (ICN 2001a, 2001b). The ICN reminds nurses of their responsibilities when faced with terrorism and bio-terrorism. These include: helping people to cope with the aftermath of terrorism, allaying public concerns and fear of bio-terrorism, identifying the feelings that nurses and others may be experiencing, assisting victims to think positively and to move to the future, and preparing nursing personnel to be effective in a crisis or emergency situation (ICN 2001b).

Nurses themselves may be the victims, survivors or citizens of a country attacked by terrorists. They may be ethically in favour of care for all, but also demonstrate patriotism for their own country. They may experience conflicting values between promoting humanism in the care of all while supporting the fighting capacity of their own army (Garfield *et al.* 2003). Negative experiences of terrorism, and the religious and cultural backgrounds of nurses, may influence their point of view on this subject. They are also human (Oulton 2001). However, nurses are foremost members of a profession that deals with the life and health of other people. Protecting life is a core value in nursing. As a pre-requisite of that value, nurses must speak out against terrorism because it contradicts the ethical principle of doing no harm.

As recent attacks were perpetuated in the name of Islam, a general overview of the role of religion and religious fundamentalism is necessary to discuss the underlying factors of Islamic fundamentalism and terrorism.

RELIGION AND FUNDAMENTALISM

Religion is a belief system that involves worship of a deity or supernatural being. Since the source of religion is divine and therefore considered indisputable, it is also naturally conservative and normative. Religion has taken on a supreme power that affects the values, morals, customs, thoughts and general behaviour patterns of people. It provides social conformity and solidarity, and thereby fosters peace and tolerance. However, religion can also catalyse conflicts and wars by providing a distinguishing character between believers and non-believers, adherents and people not adhering to its tenets. Israela Silberman *et al.* (2005) describe religion as a double-edged sword that can encourage and discourage world change, and can facilitate both violent and peaceful activism. On the one hand, religions often include values that can promote conflict resolution and peace. On the other hand, religion can provide an excellent source of legitimisation of the most violent acts, because of its power to justify morally any goal or action through sanctification (Fox 1999).

Intensive activism in the name of religion has been perpetuated throughout human history. The Crusades; the Spanish Inquisition; and the conflict between Jews and Muslims in the Middle East, Catholics and Protestants in Ireland, Muslims and Hindus in Pakistan and Bangladesh, and Christians and Muslims in the former Yugoslavia, are only some of the numerous historical acts of violence and wars (Silberman *et al.* 2005). The role of religion in encouraging peace and tolerance or aggression depends on the interpretations of the religious messages by its believers. This, in turn, defines the depth of belief and devotion of people to their religion, which orientates their world views and practices either in the direction of peace or violent action in such situations.

According to Grahame Thompson (2006), fundamentalism is an idealised religious movement that transcends cultures in its single-minded devotion to the word of God. Fundamentalists are absolutely certain about their beliefs and destinies. John Donohue (2004) defines fundamentalism as a reaction and an attempt to change the course of action. He points out that possible reactions to change may be adaptation or assimilation, withdrawal and isolation, and rejection and return to one's authentic roots to re-establish identity. Fundamentalism rejects modernity and its primary aim is to preserve the past. Fundamentalism differs from radicalism. Although they are both extremist and start out from a discontent with change, the aim of fundamentalism is to restore things and life-styles according to the past, while the orientation of radicalism is towards the future, not only maintaining the past but also changing or replacing it with religious ideals.

In recent years, it is Islamic fundamentalism that has come to be seen as a danger and something to be feared. However, fundamentalism can be a threat in all religions. The 'religions of the book' (or the 'Word') have 'an easily accessible canon which can serve as an authority . . . charter and reference point' and can, therefore, be very effective in the advance of oppositionalism (Marty 1992, p. 1). Relying on the paternal 'voice' of a God, any opposition to this tends to be expressed forcefully. Modern theology is largely based on interpretation of ancient texts, but when an interpretation is challenged as not modern or liberal enough, the 'voice' retrenches and resists. It is not difficult to see that in this context Geiko Müller-Fahrenholz (1992, p. 16), in speaking of institutional fundamentalism, also counts Stalinism, the Reagan and Bush administrations, and the Vatican, as 'characteristic examples' of reactions to world situations that have become uncontrollable. Jonathan Sacks (2003, p. 2) contends that 'the greatest single antidote to violence is *conversation*, speaking our fears, listening to the fears of others', but that 'too often in today's world, groups speak to themselves, not to one another'. Globalisation, guided by Western values of market and purchase, undermines the sense of common responsibility and cohesion that exists among local communities and, in order to maintain an ideology, the 'politics of *identity*' (Sacks 2003, p. 10) is becoming important. This is particularly evident in the present surge of Islam.

ISLAM AND ISLAMIC FUNDAMENTALISM

Islam is the second-largest world religion. The primary source of Islamic religion is the holy book, the Qur'an (Koran). The meanings of many verses in the Qur'an are often unclear. That is, the meaning of some texts or verses may be metaphorical and therefore understandable only by the clarifications of Hadith, the sayings of the Prophet Mohammed on faith and life, and the comments of Islamic scholars. Therefore, Islam has been interpreted within different meaning systems, and different groupings, such as Sunni, Shi'a, and Sufism, have their variations in religious practices (Al Sayyid 2002).

Islam is a belief system that not only covers the realm of personal faith and private life; it also provides guidance and principles for all aspects of life, from relations between individuals to business and governance, in order to establish a just society. In this context, Islam emphasises the concept of 'ummah', a community of believers regardless of their racial, national or ethnic identity. The 'ummah' can be viewed as a common consciousness and a collective Islamic identity for all Muslims (Riaz 2006). While such a religious collective identity provides a framework for moral cohesion and facilitates the interaction and collaboration of Muslims in creating social, economic and political networks in the spirit of Islamic values and ideals, it also entails religious values and ideals over plurality of rational thought, and group loyalty over individual autonomy and interests. As such, Islamic identity can provide a basis for Islamic fundamentalism. This possibility is reflected in the fact that for many Islamic movements the notion of 'ummah' is an integral part of their religious and political discourses.

However, the assumption that Islamic identity alone gives rise to fundamentalism would be misleading, because despite this collective identity, the Islamic world view and practices of Muslims around the world vary widely according to their cultural, social and ethnic diversity (Riaz 2006). There are also attempts within the Muslim world to reconstitute a liberal and market-friendly Islam or to redefine Islam in national terms to consolidate the nation-state identity. However, certain circumstances, for instance any perception of an assault on Islam, may awaken the sense of 'ummah', and Muslims may appeal to the unifying function of Islamic identity in order to react collectively. Such a reaction may inflame fundamentalist movements and Islamism. Mehdi Mozaffari (2005) points out that 'Islamic terrorism' is an immediate derivative of 'Islamism'. He argues that this term distinguishes itself from 'Islamic' by the fact that Islamic refers to a religion and a culture in existence over a millennium, whereas terrorism is a political/religious phenomenon linked to the great events of the twentieth century. He defines Islamism as a militant, antidemocratic movement, bearing a holistic vision of Islam whose final aim is the restoration of a worldwide caliphate; that is, a spiritual and political leadership of the Islamic world. From this point of view, Islamism is both a fundamentalist and radical movement, and Islamic terrorism is a violent extension of Islamism.

SOME REASONS FOR ISLAMIC FUNDAMENTALISM AND TERRORISM

The evolution of Islamic fundamentalism and the rise of terrorism did not form in a vacuum; rather they were constituted over time and have been precipitated mainly by socio-economic and political factors.

Islamic fundamentalism is a reaction to change and the new global order. Western colonialism in the ninteenth and twentieth centuries, industrialisation, nationalisation, secularism, modernisation, globalisation and the free-market economy have all contributed to the spread of Islamic fundamentalism. Globalisation has placed traditional cultures under siege because of the spread of Western culture (Wirtz 2003). This is perceived as an onslaught on less privileged people in traditional cultures and on the conservative lifestyle of many Muslims. Globalisation is not only the transmission of information and technology but also the free trade of goods, services and capital according to the neo-liberal politics enforced by the World Bank and International Monetary Fund (IMF). The 'structural adjustment' policies demanded by these institutions aggravated poverty and unemployment in developing countries by neglecting essential needs such as education, healthcare and infrastructures, because they forced governments to open their markets to international trade (Benatar *et al.* 2003; Tierney 2003).

Muslims live mainly in either very poor countries (North Africa) or in regions rich in oil reserves but under the colonialist influence of the US and Western countries. In addition, the Middle East, the region where most Muslims live, experienced social tensions and conflicts fed by poverty and unemployment. For instance, real per-capita income and consumption in the West Bank and Gaza dropped by about a third between 1999 and 2003. Individuals living in refugee camps, most of which were created in the conflict with Israel in 1948 but never demolished, are more likely to be poor than those living in urban or rural locations. The unemployment rate was 26% in 2003 (Palestinian Central Bureau of Statistics 2004). A sense of inequality and powerlessness stemming from economic decline and poverty, and alienation from the new world order forced many Muslim people to turn to Islamic fundamentalism (Silverman 2002; Cronin 2002/2003; Beeson & Bellamy 2003).

Fathali Moghaddam (2005) describes a 'staircase of terrorism' involving a metaphorical 'ground floor' and 'five higher floors'. He states that, although the vast majority of people, even when feeling deprived and unfairly treated, remains on the ground floor, some individuals climb up and are eventually recruited into terrorist organisations. It seems that poverty and negative consequences of globalisation function mainly at the ground floor, but Islamic fundamentalism can be regarded as the first step of the staircase of terrorism. However, the fact that most terrorists are from middle and well-educated classes reveals that poverty and globalisation are only part of the problem. Pete Lentini and Muhammad Bakashmar (2007) describe the following factors as contributing to the spread of Islamic fundamentalism, Islamism and Islamist terrorism: the export of Wahhabism, the strict brand of Islam found in Saudi Arabia since the beginning of the 1970s; the Iranian Islamic revolution of 1979 that served as an alternative in practice to capitalist states with liberal-democratic governments; the Soviet Union's 1979 invasion of Afghanistan and its withdrawal as a result of Muslim fighters' struggle; the proliferation of ethno-religious conflicts involving Muslims, including those in Bosnia, Kosova, Chechnya and Tajikistan; the system of Islamist training camps in Sudan and Afghanistan under Taliban, and the emergence of Al Qaeda, the international militant organisation led by Osama bin Laden.

While these factors contributed to the spread of Islamism and terrorism, these have reached their peak in recent years because of the unilateral politics of the US in the Middle East. American power has been associated with the consolidation of a particular neo-liberal order that disadvantages the developing world (Al Sayyid 2002; Silverman 2002; Beeson & Bellamy 2003). In addition, the US has assumed a biased role in the Palestinian–Israel conflict since 1967. The US provides economic and military support to Israel, but considers Palestinians fighting Israeli troops inside the occupied West Bank and Gaza as terrorists (Al Sayyid 2002; Wanandi 2002; Mazarr 2004). Keith Suter (2005) points out that there is no agreed definition of terrorism at international level. He continues: 'The practical problem is that one government's "terrorist" is another's "freedom fighter".' Most Muslims regard Palestinians as freedom fighters. The continuing Iraq war and occupation, which until the middle of 2007 has caused over 650 000 deaths, as well as torture in prisons, has triggered the anger of Islamic extremists and distorted it in the direction of violence towards the US and its allies (Al Sayyid 2002; Beeson & Bellamy 2003; Silverman 2002; Wanandi 2002). It is paradoxical that the main beneficiaries of US politics in the Middle East and the invasion of Iraq are now US-based giant oil companies and radical Islamists. The Middle East is in conflict more than ever before, and it seems that Islamic fundamentalism and terrorism may thrive by drawing increasingly on the sympathy of Muslims around the world, attracted by the 'ummah' and retrenching into its less welcomed aspects.

CONCLUDING REMARKS FOR NURSES

Terrorism is an attack on human life and health, freedom, democracy and peace. Although there are many verses in the Qur'an that strongly commend peace, the unity of all humanity and turning away from violence, Islamic terrorists prefer to

use selectively the word 'jihad' in order to justify violence and slaughter of inno-
cent people (Al Sayyid 2002). They have not only done harm to many people, but
also to the religion they believe to represent because, by abusing Islam for their
own aims, they also create a vision of Islam that appears to be militant, reactionary
and violent (Silverman 2002). As a result of such a vision, Islamic communities
and Muslim people generally have become targets of increased hostility (Hall
2004). If the chain of this hostile circle cannot be broken and the polarisation
between 'us' and 'them' continues, there will be no winners but many losers.

Terrorism must be prevented because it is destructive and unethical. However,
without considering the roots of terrorism, military and political actions will be
limited. At the same time, Islamic fundamentalism should also be better understood and addressed. There are attempts to propose a moderate Islam that is
compatible with the free-market economy as a corrective and an alternative model
to Islamic fundamentalism and radicalism. Such a model is especially supported
by European countries and the US in Turkey, a country often portrayed for
its secular, nationalist and democratic stance. However, many people believe
that moderate Islam in Turkey is only a front and will sooner or later turn into
Islamic fundamentalism, even radicalism. The increase of Qur'anic schools and
dormitories where religious ideals are imposed on the minds of students, the
controversy of the headscarf for women, an alcohol ban in public restaurants,
separating women and men in many places, and increasingly staffing official
positions with religious personnel are striking examples of the growing salience
of Islam in Turkey since the late 1990s (Onar 2006).

Islamic fundamentalism is dangerous, not only because it provides a starting
point for violent acts, but also because it is oppressive and restrictive for women,
especially in Islamic states such as Iran, Afghanistan, Saudi Arabia, Pakistan and
Sudan. Islamic fundamentalism contradicts human rights, especially women's
rights, by reinforcing the traditional male-dominated practices of beating women;
honour killings (of women who have been perceived as having brought dishonour
to their family); separating women and men in public places; obligatory veiling
and arranged marriages without taking into consideration the autonomy of
women. It fosters intolerance of religious minorities or atheists, homosexual
people, and modern and secular life-styles.

Nursing is overwhelmingly a women's profession, and unfortunately women's
professions remain undervalued by society, in particular in countries where
patriarchal cultures prevail. Nurses should therefore consider the consequences of
Islamic fundamentalism from the point of view of the status of women in society
and of the development of the nursing profession, and especially from the point
of view of their responsibilities to respect human rights.

People and communities have the right to organise their private lives in accordance with the teaching of Islam, and they have the right to participate in the political process. The political participation of Islamic parties is also a requirement of the democratisation process. However, the manner in which persons, ideological, ethnic or religious groups exercise their rights have consequences for the rights of others. Extreme religious beliefs of any kind tend to influence the political decisions and actions of their adherents when they act as officials of the state. Islam and politics cannot be separated, but Islam and the state should be institutionally separated, as is the case in many countries where religion and the state are separated. This is increasingly a requirement to ensure the rights of all citizens without any discrimination, and especially for people who want to live an Islamic life-style without any coercive enforcement by the state. It is also necessary that Islam has an educative role without being used for political or violent aims. In order to find a reasonable solution to prevent Islamic fundamentalism and terrorism, the underlying factors of Islamic terrorism must be seriously considered.

Islamic fundamentalism appeals not only as an alternative to secularism, modernism and nationalism, but also to globalisation, to the unilateral politics of the US and the EU's reluctance to confront global inequalities and political inconsistencies. Terrorism must be prevented and terrorists must not be allowed to prevail. Every country has the right to defend its land and citizens against terrorist attacks. However, international efforts should be concentrated not only on military and political issues, but also on the underlying factors that gave rise to terrorism. Terrorism is a reaction to the perception of marginalisation, disenfranchisement, and/or victimisation (Arena & Arrigo 2005). As Mazarr (2004) states, responding strategically to the threat of terrorism must mean a broad-based effort to address the sources of resentment and the psychological roots of radicalism and terrorism in the Islamic world. People everywhere, whether they are Jews, Christians, Muslims or of whatever religious persuasion, must keep in mind that we have only one Earth. We have to be very much aware of one another's existence, beliefs, and cultures and respect these. 'The ingrained attitudes of "them" and "us" are no longer tenable; the planet is too small for that. People, and nurses in particular, in developed countries have a responsibility to those in developing countries; people in developing countries need to know that they are part of a global movement towards adequate health care for everyone' (Tschudin & Schmitz 2003, p. 355). Nurses are the health professionals closest to the general public and they have the opportunity to explain the threat, causes and consequences of terrorism. They also have it in their power to advocate non-violent and more democratic ways to resolve conflicts, to relieve tensions and to demonstrate a peaceful activism. This is also our professional and ethical responsibility.

REFERENCES

Al Sayyid M. Mixed Message: the Arab and Muslim response to terrorism. *Washington Quarterly*. 2002; **25**(2): 177–90.

Arena MP, Arrigo BA. Social Psychology, Terrorism, and Identity: a preliminary re-examination of theory, culture, self, and society. *Behavioral Sciences and the Law*. 2005; **23**(4): 485–506.

Beeson, M, Bellamy AJ. Globalisation, Security and International Order After 11 September. *Australian Journal of Politics and History*. 2003; **49**(3): 339–54.

Benatar SR, Daar AS, Singer PA. Global Health Ethics: the rationale for mutual caring. *International Affairs*. 2003; **79**(1): 107–38.

Cronin AK. Behind the Curve: globalization and international terrorism. *International Security*. 2002/2003; **27**(3): 30–58.

Donohue J. Mistranslations of God: fundamentalism in the twenty-first century. *Islam and Christian-Muslim Relations*. 2004; **15**(4): 427–42.

Fox J. Do Religious Institutions Support Violence or the Status Quo? *Studies in Conflict and Terrorism*. 1999; **22**(2): 119–39.

Garfield R, Dresden E, Rafferty AM. Commentary: the evolving role of nurses in terrorism and war. *American Journal of Infection Control*. 2003; **31**(3): 163–7.

Hall JM. Marginalization and Symbolic Violence in a World of Differences: war and parallels to nursing practice. *Nursing Philosophy*. 2004; **5**(1): 41–53.

ICN. *Resources for Coping with Terrorism*. Newsroom. 2001a. Available at: http://www.icn.ch/terrorism.htm#coping (accessed 2 December 2005).

ICN. *Terrorism and Bioterrorism: nursing preparedness*. Fact Sheets, Nursing Matters. 2001b. Available from: http://www.icn.ch/matters_bio.htm (accessed 2 December 2005).

ICN. *Code of Ethics for Nurses*. Geneva: ICN; 2006.

Lentini P, Bakashmar M. Jihadist Beheading: a convergence of technology, theology, and teleology? *Studies in Conflict & Terrorism*. 2007; **30**(4): 303–25.

Marty ME. What is Fundamentalism? Theological perspectives. In: Küng H, Moltman J, editors. *Fundamentalism as an Ecumenical Challenge*. London: SCM Press; 1992. pp. 1–11.

Mazarr MJ. The Psychological Sources of Islamic Terrorism. *Policy Review*. 2004; **125**: 39–60.

Miguel-Tobal JJ, Cano-Vindel A, Gonzales-Ordi H, et al. PTSD and Depression After the Madrid March 11 Train Bombings. *Journal of Traumatic Stress*. 2006; **19**(1): 69–80.

Moghaddam FM. The Staircase to Terrorism: a psychological exploration. *American Psychologist*. 2005; **60**(2): 161–9.

Moline J, Herbert R, Nguyen N. Health Consequences of the September 11 World Trade Center Attacks: a review. *Cancer Investigation*. 2006; **24**(3): 294–301.

Mozaffari M. Bin Laden, Islamism, and Terrorism. *Society*. 2005; **42**(5): 34–42.

Müller-Fahrenholz G. What is Fundamentalism Today? Perspectives in social psychology. In: Küng H, Moltman J, editors. *Fundamentalism as an Ecumenical Challenge*. London: SCM Press; 1992. pp. 12–19.

Onar N. Kemalists, Islamists and Liberals: shifting patterns of confrontation and consensus, 2002–06. *Turkish Studies*. 2006; **8**(2): 273–88.

Oulton JA. *The Capacity to Care: an open letter from ICN's chief executive officer*. Geneva: ICN; 2001. Available at: http://www.icn.ch/openletter.pdf (accessed 10 March 2005).

Palestinian Central Bureau of Statistics and the World Bank West Bank and Gaza Office. *Poverty in the West Bank and Gaza After Three Years of Economic Crisis: deep Palestinian poverty in the midst of economic crisis.* 22 November 2004. Available from: http://siteresources. worldbank.org/INTWESTBANKGAZA/Data%20and%20Reference/20285714/ Poverty+Eng+final.pdf (accessed 9 July 2007).

Riaz H. Globalisation's Challenge to the Islamic Ummah. *Asian Journal of Social Science.* 2006; **34**(2): 311–23.

Sacks J. *The Dignity of Difference: how to avoid the clash of civilizations.* Rev. ed. London: Continuum; 2003.

Silberman I, Higgins ET, Dweck CS. Religion and World Change: violence and terrorism versus peace. *Journal of Social Issues.* 2005; **61**(4): 761–84.

Silva MC, Ludwick R. Ethics and Terrorism: September 11, 2001 and its aftermath. *Online Journal of Issues in Nursing.* 31 January 2003. Available at: www.nursingworld.org/ojin/ ethicol/ethics_11.htm (accessed 10 March 2003).

Silverman AL. Just War, Jihad, and Terrorism: a comparison of Western and Islamic norms for the use of political violence. *Journal of Church and State.* 2002; **44**(1): 73–92.

Suter K. Terrorism and International Law. *Contemporary Review.* 2005; **287**: 216–21.

Thompson GF. Exploring Sameness and Difference: fundamentalisms and future of globalization. *Globalizations.* 2006; **3**(4): 427–33.

Tierney N. Religion and the Globalization of War. In *International Conference on Globalization and Religion.* 2003, July 27–August 2; Payap University, Chiang Mai, Thailand.

Tschudin V, Schmitz C. The Impact of Conflict and War on International Nursing and Ethics. *Nursing Ethics.* 2003; **10**(4): 354–67.

United Nations. *Universal Declaration of Human Rights.* Geneva: UN; 1948.

Wanandi J. A Global Coalition Against International Terrorism. *International Security.* 2002; **26**(4): 184–9.

Wirtz JJ. Ethics and the Return to Strategy. In: Micewski ER, editor. *Civil-Military Aspects of Military Ethics.* Vol. I. Vienna: National Defense Academy; 2003. pp. 14–21.

13

Traditional indigenous health ethics in a globalising world: an American Indian perspective

Lee Anne Nichols, Judy Goforth Parker and Susan J Henly

Acknowledgement: Dr Roxanne Struthers also contributed to this manuscript. She passed away on 10 December 2006.

INTRODUCTION

Globalisation began when the first individuals left their own people to travel among others, initiating an inevitable exchange of information and customs, including those related to health and illness. Contemporary globalisation was first recognised in economics (Levitt 1983). The Internet, now accessible from classrooms and street corners, subsequently created an astronomical increase in globalisation. With globalisation, aspects of everyday life are becoming standardised around the world. These same forces are shaping health issues and transforming them from local and national to global and international concerns.

Globalisation is a worldwide occurrence. Although as Theodore Levitt (1983) pointed out, the world's needs and desires have been homogenised, that does not mean that all our cultures have blended into one. Ethics may be viewed differently in indigenous communities compared with the standard biomedical ethical perspective taught to nurses whose education is based on a Western model. Nurses may be able to apply indigenous ethical standards to health issues involving indigenous populations in their own countries. The purpose of this chapter is to explore global health ethics from an indigenous world view and to discuss how biomedical ethics may differ from what we call 'tribal ethics'.

WHO WE ARE

We are American Indian (AI) nurses and non-AI nurses, who do not present ourselves as experts in either ethics or culture, but simply as ordinary professionals who wish to explore and expand the knowledge base regarding ethics in AI communities. In AI culture, one does not speak for others so we do not speak for all nurses, particularly AI nurses. Our goal is to provide some insight and wisdom into this topic and, if other nurses choose to do so, they may learn from this discussion. Lee Anne Nichols is a Cherokee nursing scholar and researcher devoted to improving the health of American Indians; Judy Goforth Parker is a Chickasaw nursing scholar and Chickasaw legislator working to improve the health of her tribal community; and Susan Henly is a nursing scholar with many years devoted to nursing education for American Indian students and research in American Indian health. She has no tribal affiliation. We have joined together to consider the globalisation of healthcare ethics in the light of the American Indian experience.

INDIGENOUS WORLD VIEW: FROM NATIVE AMERICA

The UN recognises more than 370 million people in 70 countries as indigenous (UNPFII 2007). Across the world, indigenous peoples strive to maintain traditional homelands and sustain traditional languages, cultures, and life-ways despite dominance of larger cultures. Over 550 tribes are indigenous to the US and are recognised by the US federal government (Indian Entities 2002; Waldman 2000). Over four million people living in the US identified an affiliation with a tribal community in the last census (Bureau of Census 2002).

Indigenous people first experienced globalisation during the eras of colonialisation and nation-state building. Existence, cultural identity, and life-ways were threatened, yet traditional ways were preserved among survivors and their descendants. These traditional ways have been passed on to the next generations. Each tribe maintained its own unique rich culture, traditions, language, ceremonies, history and spirituality. Commonalities in cultural values permeate the tribes, and generally, the values most recognised are generosity, wisdom, stewardship of the Earth, humility, circularity, connectedness, cooperation, identity, honour, holism, oneness, balance, harmony, being visionary, traditionalism and planning for the future. Respect is a central value in most American Indian indigenous communities (Ambler 2003). These cultural values provide the foundation for the morals and ethics of American Indian indigenous societies where storytelling is safeguarded as a way of passing on morality and ethical reasoning from one generation to the next.

How to apply the principles of Western biomedical ethics to healthcare situations in tribal communities may be puzzling to indigenous nurses. Compared with Native ways, the reductionistic and linear principles of Western ethics may seem incongruent with practices for resolution of health dilemmas in tribal communities. At the same time, indigenous nurses recognise the need for and importance of applying Western biomedical ethics when providing quality care to both tribal and non-tribal patients.

Tom Beauchamp and James Childress (2001) define ethics as a way of understanding the morals of life. Like concepts related to research (Smith 1999), many indigenous languages do not have readily translatable words for ideas in Western bioethics. Nevertheless, the morals or ways of living are embedded in tribal oral history and passed on to the next generation *and the next and the next,* as far as the seventh.

Indigenous societies are oral societies that value respect and honour. The way of life in an indigenous community is based on traditions, prayers and ceremonies. Old knowledge received from tradition is valued over new knowledge (Moss *et al.* 2005). Most indigenous people think circularly and holistically (Garrett 1999). The indigenous American Indian world view is not unique, but is shared by many cultures and societies across the globe. In this world view, harm committed against another person, animal or the Earth is corrected by the use of prayer, spiritual practice, tradition, ceremony and the elders' wisdom. Yet, this kind of knowledge or application of ethics in nursing has largely remained unexplored.

ETHICS: A RECOVERY OF BALANCE IS NECESSARY FOR HEALING

Ethics is a general term for ways of understanding and examining the moral life (Beauchamp & Childress 2001). Morality refers to norms about right and wrong human conduct that are so widely shared that they form a stable, although usually incomplete, social consensus. Individuals learn about basic moral standards and responsibilities while growing up (Beauchamp & Childress 2001).

We observed that an Indian sense of morality of right and wrong is based on a spiritual premise that is passed orally and symbolically, and indirectly with the use of cooperation as the way to teach morality. The stories that teach about right and wrong behaviour come from 'old' knowledge (Deloria 2006). The idea of doing good and avoiding harm is a circular process. When disrespect, harm, or disharmony are committed, then prayer, ceremony and traditions are offered to the Creator to restore harmony or health.

Respect for the person is often described as the foundation of biomedical ethical behaviour (Browne 1995; Gallagher 2007). In tribal ethics, respect for everything, including the person, community, living creatures, inanimate objects and the Earth is the cornerstone of morality in the affairs of life, including health and illness (Ambler 2003).

TRADITIONAL AMERICAN INDIAN INDIGENOUS VALUES AND BELIEFS

Indigenous people follow an oral tradition; their knowledge of right and wrong or what is referred to as 'following a sacred path' is passed through their stories (Kimbrough & Drick 1991). Children in tribal communities learn about 'tribal ethics' from their elders who tell the stories and share their knowledge or wisdom. Knowledge about right and wrong is also transmitted through art, beading, baskets, dolls, weavings, drawings, jewellery, totems, clothing, carvings, dances, songs, drumming, flute playing and regalia (Indian clothing) (Henly & Moss 2007; Nichols 2004).

The Cherokees have a traditional Indian ceremony called the stomp dance. This is spiritual in nature and is closed to people outside the community (Nichols 2004). A sacred fire is lit and burns throughout the ceremony (shown in Figure 13.1). At the stomp dance, Cherokee children are taught particularly about going down the red path (bad) or the white path (good). Figure 13.2 shows a Cherokee woman in traditional dress telling of the spiritual paths by interpreting the beading on the Sacred Belts worn at the stomp dance. The script on both illustrations, written using Sequoya's syllabary, is translated as *fire* in Figure 13.1 and *belts* in Figure 13.2.

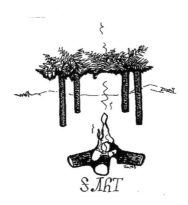

FIGURE 13.1 Sacred fire at a Cherokee stomp dance

(Reprinted with permission from SAGE Publications)

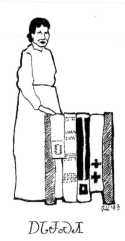

DⱢↃↄↃↃ

FIGURE 13.2 Traditional Cherokee woman with wampum belts

Tribal ethics is learned indirectly by promoting cooperation. Indigenous people are indirect in their teachings about living a moral life. Non-interference is valued (Good Tracks 1973; Greenfeld 1996; Nichols 2004, Nichols & Keltner 2005; Strong 1984; Wax & Thomas 1961) and defined as the right of the person to choose whatever type of behaviour he or she might wish to exhibit (Nichols 2004). Another family member is not allowed (or expected) to intervene, even if self-destructive behaviour is exhibited. In addition, neither can the person oppose the goals of the group.

Indigenous American Indian parents use non-interference discipline techniques to teach their children about moral behaviour. These include using adults and older children as role models, mentoring children, 'watch and listen' visual modes of learning, learning by example, ignoring misbehaviour, use of shunning, of mild rebukes, of non-verbal signals from parents or elders, and praise for good behaviours rather than punishment for wrong behaviours (Garrett 1993/1994; Nichols 2004; Nichols & Keltner 2005; Red Horse 1997; Seideman *et al.* 1996).

As tribal ethics is grounded in circular thought, tribal populations interact and think in circular ways in their interactions with the environment (Garrett 1999). In two studies conducted with indigenous nurses, seven dimensions of what the authors identified as 'native nursing' are described. The key attribute identified by the authors as relevant to native nursing is 'relationship' (Lowe & Struthers 2001; Struthers & Littlejohn 1999). It is crucial for indigenous nurses to build a relationship and connect to tribal clients prior to delivery of care. John Lowe (2002) describes the circular process of how indigenous nurses develop a oneness with Indian clients by pausing, listening, being silent and sharing informally long before any goal-directed therapeutic communication takes place. Indigenous nurses give to tribal clients so that tribal clients will feel comfortable in sharing, relating and trusting the nurses (or giving back). Nurses create the circle of care through reciprocity, and build trust to avoid violating the clients' confidence in the care being provided. In the indigenous community, caring for another is regarded as an honour and an expression of deep respect (Lowe 2002). To do otherwise would violate the tribal sense of self for indigenous clients and nurses. If tribal nurses violate the circularity of oneness created in the nurse–client relationship, nurses may feel that they have dishonoured (or behaved unethically) towards tribal clients (Greenfeld 1996; Lowe 2002).

Lee Anne Nichols (2004) described how Cherokee mothers respected their infants and used harmonious behaviours to care for their babies. Some of these behaviours included living spiritually, building a care-providing consortium, and vigilantly watching for the natural unfolding of the infant. An other study (Nichols & Keltner 2005) describes how indigenous families adjusted to having children with disabilities by using harmonious behaviours, such as caring for the child with disabilities in non-obtrusive ways. The child with a disability is valued and respected in many tribal communities (Dubray & Sanders 1999; Red Horse 1997). Annette Browne (1995) described the meaning of respect from a tribal perspective that included attributes of treating people as worthy and equal, willing to accept others, and a willingness to listen. Respect is a thread that is interwoven in an indigenous child's life. The child is taught to be respectful from birth, and is expected to be respectful of all living and non-living things; thus, by being respectful, harm to others (living and non-living) is avoided (Browne 1995; Carrese & Rhoades, 1995).

APPLICATION OF WESTERN ETHICS TO NURSING IN AN INDIGENOUS COMMUNITY: A CLINICAL ETHICAL DILEMMA

Health and illness are inexorably linked in the human experience. The transition from health to illness inevitably involves awareness or presentation of disturbing prognostic and diagnostic information which, from the Western biomedical value of truth telling, should be presented openly to support autonomy of choice in decision making. Discussion of negative medical information, such as disclosure of risk and 'bad news' and the practice of advance planning, are uncomfortable and culturally inappropriate for many indigenous patients (Carrese & Rhoades 1995; Bell 1994; Beauchamp & Childress 2001, pp. 62–3). Many indigenous nurses feel uncomfortable about 'negative information', particularly information on advance planning, with the tribal clients in their care because they fear that they might bring illness or death (harm) to their patients. They also fear negative consequences to themselves or their families if discussing taboo topics such as death and illnesses.

One way to address this ethical dilemma is to ask a traditional indigenous elder or healer from the community to conduct a talking circle with the nurses. The healer can create a sacred circle, provide prayer, make offerings to the Creator, and perform a smudging ceremony to cleanse the members of the group with smoke (Mullin *et al.* 2001). These healing techniques can protect the nurses, their families and clients from harm and are one way to ensure indigenous nurses remain on a sacred path of life and bring no harm to their patients.

GLOBAL PERSPECTIVE

In a globalising world, healthcare ethics in indigenous settings brings traditional values and practices into juxtaposition with principles and practices of Western bioethics. Creating a common voice through action is essential to providing considerate, effective and ethically justified nursing services, and to create systems of care for indigenous peoples. The International Network of Indigenous Health Knowledge and Development (INIHKD 2007) recognises similarities in disparities in health status and the systemic factors, derived from the colonialisation that created them, among the many indigenous peoples of the worlds. INIHKD advocates for linkage of received (old) traditional knowledge and contemporary health services to eliminate the burden of illness and create pathways to optimal health for indigenous peoples. The linkage of traditional values and principles of Western bioethics can be used to create balance arising from satisfactory resolution of ethical dilemmas as well.

CLOSING THOUGHTS

Ethics needs to be 'culturally sensitive, balanced, harmonious, circular, sacred, natural, holistic and unfolded with fluidity and grace' (Struthers 2001, p. 125) when applied by nurses to indigenous patients. Tribal knowledge, traditional healers, storytelling, prayer, traditions and ceremony can be applied to ethical situations to correct harm, and restore balance and harmony to tribal patients and indigenous nurses and non-indigenous nurses. Nurses can reach into the cultural wisdom and traditional knowledge of every community they serve to provide ethical care and to do no harm.

REFERENCES

Ambler M. Indigenizing our Future. *Tribal College Journal of American Indian Higher Education.* 2003; **15**(1): 8–9.

Beauchamp TL, Childress JF. *Principles of Biomedical Ethics.* 5th ed. New York: Oxford University Press; 2001.

Bell R. Prominence of Women in Navajo Healing Beliefs and Values. *Nursing & Health Care.* 1994; **15**(5): 232–40.

Browne AJ. The Meaning of Respect: A First Nations perspective. *Canadian Journal of Nursing Research.* 1995; **27**(4): 95–109.

Bureau of Census. *The American Indian and Alaska Native population: 2000: census 2000 brief.* 2002. Available at: http://www.census.gov/prod/2002pubs/c2kbr01-15.pdf (accessed 31 March 2006).

Carrese JA, Rhoades LA. Western Bioethics on the Navajo Reservation: benefit or harm. *Journal of the American Medical Association.* 1995; **274**(1): 826–9.

Deloria V Jr. *The World We Used to Live in.* Golden, CO: Fulcrum; 2006.

Dubray W, Sanders A. Interactions Between American Indian Ethnicity and Health Care. *Journal of Health & Social Policy.* 1999; **10**(4): 67–84.

Gallagher A. The Respectful Nurse. *Nursing Ethics.* 2007; **14**: 360–71.

Garrett JT. Understanding Indian Children: learning from Indian elders. *Children Today.* 1993/1994; **22**(4): 18–21.

Garrett MT. Understanding the 'Medicine' of Native American Traditional Values: an integrative review. *Counseling & Values.* 1999; **43**(2): 84–99.

Good Tracks JG. Native American Noninterference. *Social Casework.* 1973; **18**: 30–4.

Greenfeld PJ. Self, Family, and Community in White Mountain Apache Society. *Ethos.* 1996; **24**(3): 491–509.

Henly SJ, Moss MP. American Indian Health Issues. In: Boslaugh S, editor. *Encyclopedia of Epidemiology.* Thousand Oaks, CA: Sage; 2007.

Indian Entities Recognized and Eligible to Receive Services From the United States Bureau of Indian Affairs; Notice; Federal Register. 12 July 2002. Department of the Interior Bureau of Indian Affairs: National Archives and Records Administration.

INIHKD. General information. 2007. Available at: www.inihkd.org/ (accessed 27 November 2007).

Kimbrough KL, Drick CA. Traditional Indian Medicine: spiritual health process for all people. *Journal of Holistic Nursing.* 1991; **9**(1): 15–19.

Levitt T. The Globalization of Markets. *Harvard Business Review.* 1983; May–June: 1–11.

Lowe J. Balance and Harmony Through Connectedness: the intentionality of Native American nurses. *Holistic Nursing Practice.* 2002; **16**(4): 1–8.

Lowe J, Struthers R. A Conceptual Framework of Nursing in the Native American Culture. *Journal of Nursing Scholarship.* 2001; **33**(3): 279–83.

Moss M, Tibbets L, Henly SJ, *et al.* Strengthening American Indian Nurse Scientist Training Through Tradition: partnering with elders. *Journal of Cultural Diversity.* 2005; **12**(2): 50–5.

Mullin J, Lee L, Hertwig S, Silverthorn G. A Native Smudging Ceremony. *Canadian Nurse.* 2001; **97**(9): 20–2.

Nichols LA. The Infant Caring Process Among Cherokee Mothers. *Journal of Holistic Nursing.* 2004; **22**(3): 1–28.

Nichols LA, Keltner B. Indian Family Adjustment to Children With Disabilities. *American Indian and Alaska Native Mental Health Research: The Journal of the National Center.* 2005; **12**(1): 22–48. Available at: http://www.uchsc.edu/ai/ncaianmhr/journal_online.htm (accessed 15 June 2007).

Red Horse JG. Traditional American Indian Family Systems. *Families, Systems & Health.* 1997; **15**(3): 243–50.

Seideman RY, Jacobson S, Primeaux M, *et al.* Assessing American Indian Families. *American Journal of Maternal/Child Nursing.* 1996; **21**(6), 274–9.

Smith LT. *Decolonizing Methodologies: research and indigenous peoples.* London: Zed; 1999.

Strong C. Stress and Caring for Elderly Relatives: interpretations and coping strategies in an American Indian and White sample. *The Gerontologist.* 1984; **24**(3): 251–5.

Struthers R. Conducting Sacred Research: an indigenous experience. *Wicazo sa Review.* 2001; **Spring**: 125–3.

Struthers R, Littlejohn S. The Essence of Native American Nursing. *Journal of Transcultural Nursing.* 1999; **10**(2): 131–35.

UNPFII. *About UNPFII/History.* 2007. Available at: http://www.un.org/esa/socdev/unpfii/en/history.html (accessed 6 November 2007).

Waldman C. *Atlas of the North American Indian.* Rev. ed. New York: Checkmark; 2000.

Wax R, Thomas R. American Indians and White People. *Phylon.* 1961; **XXII**(4): 305–17.

14

Globalisation and imprisoned women: a challenge for nursing ethics

Anastasia A Fisher, Diane C Hatton and Anne J Davis

INTRODUCTION

The world has witnessed an unprecedented increase in the number of incarcerated women since the 1980s. Ernest Drucker (2006) notes that: 'while the United States has only 5% of the world's population, it has 25% of its prisoners' (p. 162). In fact, the US leads the world in its number of prisoners, which total over two million people. The US imprisonment rate is at its highest level in history, with more than 700 people per 100 000 of its population behind bars in 2007. Other countries have considerably lower rates of incarceration; however, the increasing trends of incarceration, especially among women, are mirrored around the world. Based on data from the International Centre for Prison Studies, Table 14.1 illustrates that the US has the most prisoners in the world, South Africa is ranked 8th, and the UK and Japan are 17th and 18th, respectively. Although it is less visible, prison growth is dramatic in the global south, where countries such as Mexico and South Africa are constructing private, US-style mega prisons (Sudbury 2002). These trends are particularly alarming given the negative impact of incarceration on health, and health disparities among poor women, especially women of colour (Australian Institute of Criminology 2005; Mauer 2003; Sudbury 2002; Freudenberg 2002; Stoller 2001).

Women prisoners are often young and poor, and experience multiple physical, mental and social health problems. They are more apt to report that before arrest they had generally poor health and enter jail or prison with serious, untreated health concerns. These include HIV, hepatitis C, TB, Methicillin-resistant *Staphylococcus aureus* (MRSA), and sexually transmitted infections (King's College London 2004; National Commission on Correctional Health Care (NCCHC) 2002). They also have higher pregnancy rates than their non-incarcerated cohorts in the general population, and histories of violence, depression, substance abuse and other mental illness (Fogel & Belyea 1999, 2001; Haywood *et al.* 2000). Ronal Braithwaite *et al.* (2005) note that 'women's medical concerns related to reproductive health and the psychosocial matters surrounding the imprisonment of single female heads of households are often overlooked' (p. 1679). These serious health and social problems present a challenge to prisons and local detention facilities that have been created, organised and managed for men, leaving the diverse needs of women forgotten and neglected (King's College London 2004; Norman & Parrish 2002).

TABLE 14.1 Number of prisoners in the US, South Africa, UK and Japan

Country	Number of prisoners	World ranking
US	2 193 798	1
South Africa	160 198	8
UK	80 316	17
Japan	79 052	18

International Centre for Prison Studies (2007)

It is estimated that two-thirds of women prisoners are mothers to minor children, yet many are geographically isolated into the few limited facilities that incarcerate women. In some countries there is only one women's prison and all the women prisoners from the entire country are held there, even though it may be many hours' or days' travel away from the women's homes and families (King's College London 2004, p. 3). This results in separation from families, legal and community resources, and makes contact with children more difficult (Fernandez 2007). In addition, women have multiple housing needs, often experiencing numerous episodes of homelessness prior to incarceration. Women also are from communities of poverty, with limited access to resources and education. Almost all women prisoners will eventually return to their communities, therefore not only do prisoners experience a myriad of health problems while incarcerated, they return to communities with untreated and serious health problems that place a substantial burden on already financially stressed healthcare systems (Freudenberg *et al.* 2005; NCCHC 2002).

The infrastructures of prisons and local detention facilities contribute to the challenges for delivery of healthcare. Local detention facilities represent a particular challenge for healthcare, in part because of their more limited funding and shorter sentences: less than one year and sometimes only a few days. Some health problems result from the very conditions of incarceration. In a study of women's healthcare in California state prisons, Nancy Stoller (2003) found the most common problems to be iatrogenic, i.e. 'those events in which medical errors in treatment . . . were clearly documented in the file as causing further health problems' (p. 2266–7). Yet, these detention facilities also present an opportunity to provide quality screening and preventive care, as well as appropriate follow-up treatment to a population at risk for negative health outcomes (Freudenberg 2002; Magee *et al.* 2005).

GLOBALISATION AND THE EXPLOSION IN WOMEN'S IMPRISONMENT

Traditionally, women who are incarcerated are viewed as flawed individuals whose personal biographies are filled with evidence of family dysfunction; childhood abuses; school, economic and relationship failures; and drug and alcohol addiction. Incarceration is often viewed as a natural outcome of these individual focused behaviours. While it is often the case that individuals who are imprisoned experience severe life events, these individual behaviours are inadequate to explain the escalation in worldwide incarceration rates. Roy Walmsley reveals: 'It is easy to assume that increases in incarceration rates are due chiefly to higher crime rates; however, more often they are the result of new laws, concerned communities, and politicians eager to show they are tough on crime' (2007, p. 30).

Globalisation offers another perspective on incarceration from that typically found in the literature that emphasises individual behaviour. Julia Sudbury (2005) suggests that the mass imprisonment of women is intimately connected to global capitalism, neoliberal politics, and US economic and military dominance. Transnational practices, shifting cross-border migration patterns, and changing trade agreements have altered women's lives and their economic opportunities. Around the world, changes in the law have expanded the range of activities and conditions punishable by criminal justice, have imposed more punishment for previously criminalised behaviours, and have treated women who serve their sentences more punitively. Social problems, such as mental illness or poverty, were once dealt with by offering a set of public and privatised services. Although systems to address these problems have been inadequate, they were nonetheless designed to address the problems. Today, services are dramatically reduced and the individual behaviours are being criminalised instead. Thus, persons who are mentally ill or poor are ending up in prison and local detention facilities whose systems are not designed or equipped to address these and other health problems and, in fact, make them worse.

In addition to changes in the law, globalisation also looks to the political economy of prisons to explain the trend towards mass incarceration. Joel Dyer (2000) notes: 'prisons involve multiple stakeholders in both the public and private sector who participate in and benefit from the shift from a rehabilitative model to a "tough on crime" culture' (p. 4). Prisons are big business and the global prison boom is an outcome of public policy and private greed, rather than individual failings (Dyer 2000). 'Spiraling incarceration rates, rampant overcrowding, and systemic human rights violations are common features of women's prisons from Lagos to Los Angeles' (Sudbury 2005, p. xiv).

HUMAN RIGHTS

The complex idea of human rights comes from the basic ethical principle of justice, and has various definitions. Anne Davis (forthcoming) defines human rights as those held by all persons equally, universally and forever. They are inalienable, indivisible and interdependent. Human rights are those basic standards without which people cannot live in dignity. To violate someone's human rights is to treat that person as though she or he were not a human being. To advocate for human rights is to demand that the human dignity of all people be respected. The most fundamental legal definition of human rights is: the basic rights and freedoms, to which all humans are entitled, often held to include the right to life and liberty, freedom of thought and expression, and equality before the law (Mann et al. 1999). Sophia Gruskin et al. (2005) note that fundamental to definitions of human rights is their articulation of the role of the state towards the individual and the role of the individual in the state, including civil, political, economic, social and cultural rights. At times, all of these rights are subsumed under the larger category of human rights.

HUMAN RIGHTS AND HEALTH

Jonathan Mann et al. (1999) were among the first to make an explicit link between health and human rights. Three distinct relationships have been identified. The first concerns the impact of health policies, programmes and practices on human rights. The second is based on the understanding that violations of human rights impact on health. Thirdly, the promotion and protection of human rights and promotion and protection of health are intrinsically linked. This final relationship really suggests that health and human rights are different sides of the same coin and that when talking about one we are talking about the other.

International recognition of the right to health took form in the preamble to the 1946 constitution of the WHO, which affirms: 'The enjoyment of the highest attainable standard of health is one of the fundamental rights of every human being without distinction of race, religion, political belief, economic or social condition' (WHO 1946). The Universal Declaration of Human Rights affirms 'everyone's right to a standard of living adequate for the health and well-being of himself and his family, including food, clothing, housing and medical care and necessary social services, and the right to security in the event of unemployment, sickness, disability, widowhood, old age or other lack of livelihood in circumstances beyond his control' (Marks 2004, p. 37). The Declaration of Alma Ata of 1978 affirmed health as a fundamental human right (Marks 2004).

HUMAN RIGHTS AND INCARCERATED PERSONS

An extraordinary amount of attention has been devoted to the human rights of prisoners, with over 23 million websites focused on rights and prisoners. According to Amnesty International (1999), many human-rights requirements related to incarcerated persons are contained in standards that have been adopted by the international community, but are not in the form of treaties. Although these standards are not technically legal treaties, they have the moral force of having been negotiated by governments, and of having been adopted by political bodies such as the UN General Assembly, often by consensus. While it is outside the scope of this chapter to review these standards, several international treaties that protect the rights of persons deprived of their liberty need to be mentioned: The International Covenant on Civil and Political Rights (ICCPR); Convention against Torture and Other Cruel, Inhuman or Degrading Treatment or Punishment (Convention against Torture); Convention on the Elimination of All Forms of Discrimination Against Women (CEDAW); and International Convention on the Elimination of All Forms of Racial Discrimination (CERD) (*see also* Chapter 6). 'The US, having made significant contributions to the development of these key international standards of human rights, remains reluctant to ratify key human rights treaties, does not implement key elements of the treaties it has ratified and has refused to permit persons within the US from bringing complaints about potential human rights violations to international monitoring bodies' (Amnesty International 1999, p. 2).

Stephen Marks (2004) notes that the First UN Congress held in 1955 on the prevention of Crime and the Treatment of Offenders adopted a set of minimum standards for the treatment of prisoners. This document establishes numerous principles, including that 'medical staff shall see and examine every prisoner as soon as possible after his admission and thereafter as necessary, with a view to the discovery of physical or mental illness and the taking of all necessary measure' (Marks 2004, p. 24). The UN Body of Principles for the Protection of All Persons under Any Form of Detention or Imprisonment (Body of Principles), adopted in 1988, contains an authoritative set of Internationally recognised minimum standards on the treatment of prisoners, including a requirement that incarcerated people be given medical care and treatment free of charge (UN 1988).

The Supreme Court of the US in Estelle *v* Gamble (1976) mandated health-care for prisoners, recognising indifference to their serious health problems as a violation of the Eighth Amendment of the US Constitution, prohibiting cruel and unusual punishment. Yet violations of the human rights of women prisoners in the US continue. Amnesty International documented significant differences between the rights of women set forth in international standards and federal and state laws in the US; for example, requirements that women prisoners be supervised by female custody staff. In contrast, under US laws, Amnesty International (1999) and Stoller (2001) note that in many jurisdictions a male guard may watch over a woman while she is dressing, showering or using the toilet. He may also touch her body during searches for contraband.

Ethics, as a branch of philosophy, deals primarily with defining morally good actions. As nurses, we encounter ethics as descriptions of or prescriptions for moral behaviour toward patients. Davis *et al.* (1997) and Cheryl Easley *et al.* (2001) indicate that these ethical mandates are often codified by professional organisations, and serve as a guide to decision making and action in specific practice situations. In addition, Easley *et al.* (2001) consider human rights and ethics to result from moral judgement about good behaviour, but in the form of mutually agreed upon norms articulating the just claims of individuals and the related obligations of the state. The universality of human rights claims derive from the agreement of practically all states to be bound by them, rather than rely on human nature.

THE NURSING PERSPECTIVE

Historically, the provision of healthcare in prisons and local detention facilities has been problematic, but the unprecedented number of imprisoned women worldwide has created a crisis. Cindy Peternelj-Taylor (2005) suggests that nurses, as the largest group of healthcare professionals practising in jails and prisons, have an opportunity to influence the health of the people in their care. However, to provide quality care, nurses must often take 'heroic action to surmount institutional obstacles to what might be normal activity in a civilian setting' (Stoller 2003, p. 2271). Contributing to the challenges of providing healthcare to prisoners is the problem of stigma. Katherine Maeve and Michael Vaughn (2001) note that working in prisons and local detention facilities is stigmatising to professionals. Professional stigma isolates those working in these facilities and makes it possible for national and international nursing leaders to view the issues of prison healthcare and the nurses working in these settings as separate, rather than part of the larger dialogue on healthcare. It is no surprise, therefore, that problems of negligent care in prisons and local detention facilities continue (Amnesty International 1999; Warren 2006).

The responsibilities of nursing to incarcerated persons/women are articulated in national and international documents. The ICN asserts that: 'prisoners and detainees have the right to health care and humane treatment' (Marks 2004, p. 31). In the Declaration of Prison Health as Part of Public Health, the WHO takes the position that 'the act of depriving a person of his or her liberty always entails a duty of care which calls for effective methods of presentation, screening and treatment' (Marks 2004, p. 30). While these documents clearly define the standards, in many cases they are not implemented and, in fact, neglect is well documented. For example, healthcare operations in California's prisons have drawn considerable media attention, as well as claims of healthcare incompetence and neglect. These conditions, Jennifer Warren (2006) notes, have led a federal judge to place the state's prison healthcare operations under a federal receivership. The crisis in prison healthcare, in spite of international and national documents proclaiming prisoners' right to healthcare and humane treatment, raises issues of social justice for nursing.

Nursing has a long tradition of advocating for social justice and human rights, but some influential nurses – such as Betty Bekemeier and Patricia Butterfield (2005) and Joyce Fitzpatrick (2003) – have suggested that we have abandoned concern for society in favour of care of the individual patient. Much of the nursing ethics literature dealing with practice in 'correctional' facilities discusses such politically charged and widely publicised issues as nurses' participation in prisoner execution. While this is clearly a significant issue, the day-to-day ethical challenges and human rights violations that impact on nurses' work in prisons and local detention facilities are largely ignored. Thus, the literature's preoccupation with 'back-end' issues, such as the nurse's role in lethal injections, overlooks the debate on what Nicolas Freudenberg et al. (2005) call the 'front-end' concerns, such as who goes to jail, how their healthcare needs are met, and what happens when they come home; these concerns are just as compelling. Maeve and Vaughan (2001) raise an even more fundamental issue with their claim 'that the most basic ethical problem for nurses working in prison is whether prisoner healthcare is a right at all' (p. 50). While we believe that prisoners deserve quality healthcare and that the state has an obligation to provide that care, we also recognise that there is little debate and dialogue among nurses about this and other prison health-care issues. We end this chapter with a series of recommendations, influenced by the global perspective on women's imprisonment, that are designed to stimulate thoughtful discussion about the health of imprisoned women and the policies that place women at risk of incarceration, as well as nursing's place in the social justice and human rights arena.

IMPLICATIONS FOR NURSING ETHICS

We recommend the use of a global perspective, with its broader lens, to shape a new debate regarding incarceration around the world. This perspective focuses nursing's social justice obligation to affect policies that reduce the burdens women experience disproportionately and that contribute to increased risk of imprisonment. We end this chapter with several strategies that focus on nursing's social justice obligations: strategies based on our belief that the health of women prisoners must be considered a mainstream topic in nursing rather than a subject of interest only to those who work in prisons or local detention facilities. To accomplish the goals of increasing awareness about and taking action to improve the health of women prisoners, we see an important role for nursing educators, practitioners and researchers.

Educators

We believe that nursing educators have a responsibility to include content in curricula about human rights, social determinants of health and policies that impact the health of women, and how these contribute to or reduce the opportunity for incarceration. The ICN's Girl Child Program is an example of an important international initiative to improve the lives of young girls, thereby reducing the risk of incarceration later in life (ICN 2000). This and other programmes can inform nursing curricula around the world.

Prison nurses

Nurses working in prisons and local detention facilities, either providing direct care to individuals or serving as administrators in these extremely complex organisations, have opportunity and responsibility to improve the health of women prisoners. While we acknowledge the difficulty of this work, we encourage nurses who practise in prisons and local detention facilities to examine and implement aspects of model programmes for healthcare delivery in these unique settings. Programmes such as the Health in Prison Project (HIPP) and the National Health Services in the UK are two examples.

Nurse researchers

We also encourage nurse researchers to conduct studies that focus on policies impacting on the health of imprisoned women and their children, including investigations on limited access to services, homelessness, and violence and substance abuse. Such life conditions are frequently experienced by imprisoned women. We are currently conducting this type of project in our examination of the impact of the prisoner co-payment for healthcare policy on women's health

(Fisher & Hatton 2007). Through this project and research by others, nurse scientists can examine how policies impact on the health of women prisoners, exacerbate their health disparities, and violate their human rights.

International nursing leaders

The goal to reduce the health disparities and human rights violations associated with mass imprisonment is lofty, and requires national and international nursing action. We encourage nursing leaders around the world to make health of women prisoners a priority initiative in order to increase visibility of and education about this subject; to publish relevant articles in 'mainstream' nursing journals and to solicit manuscripts for special topic issues; and to present papers on the subject in national and international conferences. By increasing awareness and taking political action to challenge policies that are harmful to the health of women prisoners, nurses can help to shape an international debate and add their collective force to those advocates who are demanding alternatives to incarceration.

CONCLUSION

In this chapter, we outline the relevant health issues of incarcerated women around the world, the global perspective on incarceration, human rights documents acknowledging health as a human right and the challenges to nursing ethics debates. We note that the nursing ethics literature on incarceration has focused generally on politically charged issues, such as the role of nurses in prisoner execution, rather than the everyday human rights violations that characterise their work in prisons and local detention facilities. We challenge nurses to move from a perspective that holds concern for individual patients as central to a position that attends to the larger macro-social policies that impact incarceration. We believe that nursing should care deeply about prisoners' welfare, because as Norvall Morris and David Rothman (1995) have said: 'prisoners are ourselves writ large or small. And, as such, they should not be subjected to suffering exceeding fair expiation for the crimes for which they have been convicted' (p. xiii).

REFERENCES

Amnesty International. *Not Part of My Sentence: violations of the human rights of women in custody.* 1999. Available at: http://web.amnesty.org/library/print/ENGAMR510011999 (accessed 7 June 2005).

Australian Institute of Criminology. *Women and Crime: female prisoner statistics.* 2005. Available at: http://www.aic.gov.au/topics/women/stats/corrections.html (accessed 1 August 2005).

Bekemeier B, Butterfield P. Unreconciled Inconsistencies: a critical review of the concept of social justice in three national nursing documents. *Advances in Nursing Science.* 2005; **28**(2): 152–62.

Braithwaite RL, Treadwell HM, Arriola KRJ. Health Disparities and Incarcerated Women: a population ignored. *American Journal of Public Health.* 2005; **95**(10): 1679–81.

Davis AJ. The On-going Struggle for Ethical Ideals: justice and human rights. In: Hatton DC, Fisher AA, editors. *Incarcerated Women: justice and health for an international excluded population.* Abingdon: Radcliffe Publishing; (forthcoming).

Davis AJ, Aroskar MA, Liaschenko J, Drought TS. *Ethical Dilemmas and Nursing Practice.* 4th ed. Stamford, CT: Appleton & Lange; 1997.

Drucker EM. Incarcerated People. In: Levy BS, Sidel VW, editors. *Social Injustice and Public Health.* New York: Oxford University Press; 2006. pp. 161–75.

Dyer J. *The Perpetual Prisoner Machine: how America profits from crime.* Boulder, CO: Westview Press; 2000.

Easley CE, Marks SP, Russell ME. The Challenge and Place of International Human Rights in Public Health. *American Journal of Public Health.* 2001; **91**(12), 1922–25.

Estelle *v* Gamble, 429 US 97 (1976). Available at: http://www.oyez.org/cases/1970-1979/1976/1976_75_929 (accessed 4 May 2008).

Fernandez E. Visiting Mom in Prison. *San Francisco Chronicle,* 14 May 2007. Available at: http://www.sfgate.com/cgi-bin/article.cgi?f=/c/a/2007/05/14/MNGI7PQA161.DTL (accessed 18 August 2007).

Fisher A, Hatton D. *Co-payment Policy: impact on the health of women prisoners.* Paper presented at the American Public Health Association Annual Meeting, Washington DC, 3–7 November 2007.

Fitzpatrick JJ. Social Justice, Human Rights and Nursing Education. *Nursing Education Perspectives.* 2003; **24**(2): 65–7.

Fogel CI, Beylea M. The Lives of Incarcerated Women: violence, substance abuse, and at risk of HIV. *Journal of the Association of Nurses in AIDS Care.* 1999; **10**(6): 66–74.

Fogel CI, Beylea M. Psychological Risk Factors in Pregnant Inmates; a challenge for nursing. *MCN: American Journal of Maternal Child Nursing.* 2001; **26**(1): 10–16.

Freudenberg N. Adverse Effects of US Jail and Prison Policies on the Health and Well-being of Women of Colour. *American Journal of Public Health.* 2002; **92**(12): 1895–9.

Freudenberg N, Daniels J, Crum M, *et al.* Coming Home From Jail: the social and health consequences of community re-entry for women, male adolescents, and their families and communities. *American Journal of Public Health.* 2005; **95**(10): 1725–36.

Gruskin S, Grodin MA, Annas GJ, Marks SP. *Perspectives on Health and Human Rights.* New York: Routledge; 2005.

Haywood TW, Kravitz HM, Goldman LB, Freeman A. Characteristics of Women in Jail and Treatment Options. *Behavior Modification.* 2000; **24**(3): 307–24.

ICN. *ICN on the Girl Child.* 2000. Available at: http://www.icn.ch/matters_girlchild.htm (accessed 23 August 2007).

International Centre for Prison Studies. 2007. Available at: http://www.kcl.ac.uk/depsta/rel/icps/worldbrief/world_brief.html (accessed 28 July 2007).

King's College London. *Reforming Women's Prisons.* Guidance Note 13. 2004. International Centre for Prison Studies. Available at: www.kcl.ac.uk/depsta/rel/icpslgn-13-womens-prisons.pdf (accessed 9 May 2006).

Maeve MK, Vaughn MS. Nursing with Prisoners: the practice of caring, forensic nursing or penal harm nursing? *Advances in Nursing Science.* 2001; **24**(2), 47–64.

Magee CG, Hult JR, Turalba R, McMillan S. Preventive Care for Women in Prison: a qualitative community health assessment of the Papanicolaou test and follow-up treatment at a California state women's prison. *American Journal of Public Health.* 2005; **95**(10): 1712–17.

Mann J, Gostin L, Gruskin, S, *et al.* Health and Human Rights. In: Mann JM, Gruskin S, Grodin MA, Annas GJ, editors. *Health and Human Rights: a reader.* New York: Routledge; 1999. pp. 7–20.

Marks S. *Health and Human Rights: basic international documents.* Cambridge, MA: Harvard University Press; 2004.

Mauer M. *Comparative International Rates of Incarceration: an examination of causes and trends.* 2003. Available at: http://www.sentencingproject.org/pdfs/pub9036.pdf (accessed 1 August 2005).

Morris N, Rothman D. *The Oxford History of the Prison: the practice of punishment in western society.* New York: Oxford University Press; 1995.

NCCHC. March 2002. *The Health Status of Soon to be Released Inmates: a report to Congress.* Available at: http://www.ncchc.org/stbr/Volume1/Health%20Status%20(vol%201) (accessed 11 April 2003).

Norman AE, Parrish AA. *Prison Nursing.* Oxford: Blackwell Science Ltd; 2002.

Peternelj-Taylor C. Mental Health Promotion in Forensic and Correctional Environments. *Journal of Psychosocial Nursing and Mental Health Services.* 2005; **43**(9): 8–9.

Stoller N. Improving Access to Health Care for California's Women Prisoners. California Program on Access to Care, California Policy Research Center, University of California, 1–173. 2001. Available at: http://www.ucop.edu/cprc/stollerpaper.pdf (accessed 25 May 2005).

Stoller N. Space, Place and Movement as Aspects of Health Care in Three Women's Prisons. *Social Science and Medicine.* 2003; **56**(11): 2263–75.

Sudbury J. Celling Black Bodies: black women in the global prison industrial complex. *Feminist Review.* 2002; **70**: 57–74.

Sudbury J. *Global Lockdown: race, gender, and the prison-industrial complex.* New York: Routledge; 2005.

UN. *Body of Principles for the Protection of All Persons under Any Form of Detention or Imprisonment.* 1988. Available at: http://www.unhchr.ch/html/menu3/b/h_comp36.htm (accessed 15 May 2006).

Walmsley, R. Prison Planet. *Foreign Policy.* 2007; **160**: 30–1.

Warren J. Judge Steps up Pressure on State Prison System. *Los Angeles Times,* 15 March 2006. Available at: http://www.latimes.com/news/local/la-me-prisons15mar15,1,7396448.story (accessed 28 March 2006).

WHO. Constitution, 22 July 1946. Available at: http://www.yale.edu/lawweb/avalon/decade/decad051.htm (accessed 20 May 2006).

SECTION 5

Nurse education

15

In whose best interest? Balancing registered nurse competence standards with the need for more nurses and ethical treatment for immigrant nurses

Elizabeth Niven

INTRODUCTION

At its best, the globalisation of nursing may be envisaged as the free movement of registered nurses from one country to another, with a registration universally accepted and employment situations open to any registered nurse. In reality, there are many barriers to this utopian scenario. Except for a few instances, for example, between Australia and New Zealand, there is no real reciprocity of registration. The Caribbean Commonwealth countries implemented a regional examination in 1990 as the first rationale for reciprocity among the countries of the region (Reid 2000). Most countries, however, including those in the EU, continue to assess the education and practice of foreign-registered nurses in order to judge whether they should be granted registration status in their new country. Clearly there must be a high degree of congruity in education, clinical preparation, clinical experience and social structure before automatic reciprocal registration is agreed. This chapter discusses the situation for those nurses immigrating to New Zealand whose registration is accepted, but whose competence must still be evaluated through a course that includes both instruction and clinical assessment. Other countries face similar challenges, and the New Zealand experience may provide information to both nurses and registration bodies.

INTERNATIONAL TRENDS

A shift from a simple renewal of registration to systems that focus on the competence of health professionals is evident in many countries, beginning with Canada (Nelson & Purkis 2004) and the UK in the early 1990s (NMC 2001) and since then in various individual states in the US (Smolenski 2005). These changes have not been without challenge in relation to such elements as how well reflection can actually measure competence (Smolenski 2005) and the issue of random audit (Australian Nursing Federation (ANF) 2002). In New Zealand, the Health Practitioner Competence Assurance Act 2003 requires professional boards to be established for a range of health professionals, and for systems for assessment of competence to be established. It is not surprising, then, to see growing concerns about the clinical performance and competence of immigrant nurses (Mulrooney 2005; Pearson 2005). Processes to measure competence of immigrant nurses are appearing among national registration bodies (NMC 2007). A UK employer found that the new requirements created barriers to the employment of immigrant nurses (Mulrooney 2005), but the registration bodies defended the actions as being for the public good (Turton 2005).

NURSES ENTERING AND LEAVING NEW ZEALAND

The standard of nursing education and practice has been important in New Zealand for more than 100 years. From 1870 the new Nightingale nurses were invited to help set up training schools, and in 1901 the world's first registration act for nurses was introduced (Papps & Kilpatrick 2002).

Today, immigrant nurses are still welcomed. New registrations for immigrant nurses can exceed those from nursing schools in New Zealand in some years. The 2004–05 figures show that of a total of 2938 new registrations, 1612 (more than half) were overseas registered nurses (Clark 2006). It is important that these immigrant nurses are welcomed appropriately and prepared for nursing practice in their new country of residence.

NEW ZEALAND NURSES OVERSEAS

While the world continues to struggle with the challenge of nurse migration, New Zealand is in the paradoxical position of being both an exporter and an importer of nurses. As a young and developing country we welcome new immigrants, particularly those with skills the country needs. The 2006 census showed the proportion of the population born overseas as 23% (Spoonley 2007), supporting the argument that our nurse population should reflect the diversity of the larger population.

New Zealanders also have a strong tradition of 'doing the OE' (overseas experience), in which young, and more recently, not so young, people spend time living and working abroad. Nurses are among the people who travel, particularly to those countries that offer recognition of their qualifications. The majority of these nurses return to New Zealand with valuable experience that adds to the quality of their practice, and with the knowledge that they have made a contribution to the delivery of health in another country.

This means that a number of nurses who undertook their education in New Zealand have firsthand experience of seeking recognition of their registration in another country, and also of the challenges of integrating into an unfamiliar working environment. Such experiences range from excellent periods of work that are beneficial to the host country (Webby & Barnett 2005) to meeting ineptitude that resulted in negative accounts (Farag 2006), which can benefit neither party. Changing requirements also make international nursing registration and working difficult. For example, in the 1960s, '70s and '80s nurses could gain registration in the UK quite readily. Now, if New Zealand nurses want to work in the UK, they have to undertake an English language test and practise under supervision.

This begs the question: what restrictions to registration are fair and reasonable, and what restrictions may be unreasonable, or even unethical? New Zealanders, Canadians, Australians and US citizens use English as their first language: their education is – except in Quebec – undertaken in English; their nursing practice uses English. Why then should they have to take an English test? We might therefore just as reasonably ask nurses from the UK to take an English language test on arrival in New Zealand. However, New Zealand, too, has increasingly stringent requirements. How do these appear to prospective immigrant nurses?

OVERSEAS NURSES IN NEW ZEALAND

Nurses whose first registration is in overseas countries will request acceptance of their registration from the Nursing Council, New Zealand's official registration body for nurses. The majority of these nurses will have straightforward recognition of their education and experience, but a small number will be required to undertake further instruction, assessment of competence, or both. Their experiences form the central discussion of this chapter.

WHY IS NEW ZEALAND ACCEPTING FOREIGN NURSES?

As in most other countries, there is a shortage of nurses in New Zealand. Pay, conditions of work and social respect are all issues that reduce entry to nursing schools and discourage those in the profession from staying. In addition, frequent health restructuring commonly removes higher levels of nursing posts, thus diminishing career development prospects. An ICN press release (2006) reporting a two-year study on the worldwide nursing shortages identified five priority areas to address the problem: funding, workforce policy, positive practice environments, recruitment and retention, and nursing leadership. This confirms that the New Zealand experience is common.

MIGRANT NURSES COMING TO NEW ZEALAND

The ethical issues relating to migration of nurses are many. I address here the concerns about how nurses are prepared and accepted into their profession in a new country. Immigrant nurses who apply for registration to the Nursing Council of New Zealand (NCNZ) fall into three general categories: those not accepted, those accepted without requirements, and those accepted subject to successful competence assessment. The **2004** and 2006 numbers show (Cassie 2006) that New Zealand still hires most of its overseas nurses from the UK (**829**; 704). Other sources are the Philippines (**147**; 146), Australia (**136**; 124), South Africa (**105**; 47), Zimbabwe (**77**; 102), US (**75**; 29) and India (**55**; 90). Smaller numbers came from many other countries, including 10 nurses from China.

The majority of these nurses will not be asked to complete a competence assessment course, and will undertake the orientation period offered by their new employer. Such orientation will normally include some introduction to New Zealand culture and the founding document of the country, the Treaty of Waitangi. New Zealand nurses value culturally sensitive nursing practice, which has developed from partnerships with the first people of the land (Maori) and those who arrived subsequently, collectively called by the Maori people Tau Iwi, meaning those who are not the first people of the land. In 2004, the then professional adviser of the New Zealand Nurses Organisation, Faith Roberts, herself an immigrant nurse from the UK, recommended that all overseas nurses should undertake compulsory cultural safety training (O'Connor 2004).

COMPETENCE ASSESSMENT COURSE

It should be noted that this training course does not assess the applicants' nursing knowledge in relation to their acceptance as registered nurses; that has been assessed by the NCNZ before they are approved to enter the course. The course measures the competence of the new nurses to practise in the New Zealand setting. While the length of the course may vary a little, depending on the recommendation of the NCNZ about the applicants' individual requirements, it is generally eight weeks, and consists of a mix of theory and supervised clinical experience.

COMPETENCE ASSESSMENT COURSES FOR MIGRANT NURSES

Specific courses have been offered at many institutions since 1997. They require constant review and update for three key reasons. Firstly, the criteria set by the NCNZ have developed and changed over time. For example, in the earlier years English language tests could be the institution's own tests, but now applicants must show passes of specified levels in one of three approved tests before they enter any course. In addition the NCNZ now undertakes pre-screening tests, such as police records, saving the institution time and costs. Secondly, the pattern of immigration fluctuates over time; currently most foreign graduates entering a competence assessment programme are from India and the Philippines; in the late 1990s they were mostly from China, Taiwan and Korea; in 2000 there were significant numbers of nurses from Eastern Europe (Cassie 2006). Those who deliver the courses must remain aware of the backgrounds from which the registered nurses come. In some situations, the nurses are the forerunners for an emigrating family group; such a responsibility can be heavy and many nurses experience a high level of anxiety as a consequence. The third need for continual review relates to the environment in which nursing takes place. The health sector changes continually and the new nurses need the most up-to-date information.

WHY ASSESS COMPETENCE IF THE NURSES' EDUCATION IS 'EQUIVALENT'?

Each application from overseas-registered nurses is evaluated individually. The majority of applicants have many years of clinical practice, they show the required level of English language and their education is judged as 'equivalent'. Given that most of the nurses who undertake a competence assessment course are eventually fully accepted onto the New Zealand register, would it not be fairer to omit this expensive phase? After all, employers offer orientation to the workplace, most offer some introduction to New Zealand society, and immigration processes offer information about settling in their new country.

The NCNZ has a statutory obligation to ensure that all nurses accepted onto the register are competent to practise. In situations where the NCNZ judges that the information provided in relation to competence is insufficient for it to evaluate competence, it must request assessment. The judgement is that competence is likely but not currently evident, and must be demonstrated in the New Zealand setting. The aim of the course is to provide information and support for these overseas-registered nurses so that they can demonstrate their competence.

Could such assessment take place through a simple and prescribed orientation to a workplace and routine performance reviews? At this point it is necessary to acknowledge that the contexts in which nursing takes place can vary considerably. Where there are major differences between the old and the new society in language, culture, social structure, religion, the provision of healthcare and the status of nurses, the ability to make a fair assessment of competence is problematic. Therefore, it is fair for applicants whose competence is not fully evident in their application to have the benefit of the best possible circumstances for assessment.

HOW WELL DO THE COURSES WORK?

The success rating of courses is high; nurses have made a substantial investment and they are highly committed to succeed. Occasionally a nurse will have a real knowledge deficit and simply have insufficient nursing knowledge to undertake safe nursing practice. Very occasionally a nurse will be unable to adapt to the new social expectations of the new country. Generally, such nurses will leave the course; but sometimes the institution is unable to confirm to the NCNZ that competence to practise in the New Zealand setting has been shown. Assessment is multi-factorial, in that short tests, clinical evaluation, oral discussions and personal reflections all contribute to the final decision. Once full registration has been confirmed by the NCNZ, most registered nurses integrate well into New Zealand society.

FORMAL EVALUATION OF THE EFFECTIVENESS OF ONE PROGRAMME

The programme director of one overseas-registered nurse course, Kath Seton, undertook a study on the first year of clinical experiences of nurses graduating from the programme (Seton 2004).

The findings show that nurses come to New Zealand with individual and different ideas of what nursing practice entails, and what professional nursing means to them. They experienced some degree of culture shock as they made a personal and a professional adaptation to nursing in New Zealand. Key issues were communication and workplace culture. Although a reasonably high level of English is required for entry to practice (now 7.0 International English Language Test System (IELTS)), the new nurses still met barriers of local accents, colloquial language, abbreviations and non-verbal communication. In relation to communication, the nurses had differing experiences and views. Some nurses found the idea of therapeutic communication in non-mental health settings new to them; others judged New Zealand nurses as non-caring when they did not spend time communicating with patients. These comments illustrate the potential for both similarity and difference that naturally occur in nursing settings.

Seton observed that competence and communication are linked in the clinical experience of these new nurses. When they could not understand the subtleties of meaning they were concerned that they appeared not competent as registered nurses. Breakdowns in communication were also commonly the cause of bad experiences with other staff, with patients and with relatives. The need to show competence during the assessment is paramount in the minds of the nurses, and any event that could show a lack of competence would be likely to increase anxiety and further hamper communication.

Professional adaptation was key to long-term settling in at the workplace. Nursing care is delivered worldwide in a variety of ways, such as task-oriented, team nursing, primary care nursing and key workers. Professional relationships also vary, from hierarchical and formal, to more friendly and casual. The registered nurses in Seton's study all had English as their second language, and came from a variety of countries and cultures. The boundaries between the care provided by registered nurses, caregivers or nurse assistants, family members and medical staff differ from country to country, and may also differ in settings within a single country. For example, direct patient care in New Zealand is provided by both registered nurses and nursing assistants. Family members are welcome to provide personal care, but are not expected to do so.

For many of the nurses in Seton's study, direct patient care was not something they had practised. In New Zealand, nurses are expected to plan and manage nursing care; for example, making decisions about wound management. For some nurses such responsibility was new; for others it was familiar practice. Gradual adjustment to these different practices is shown in the reflective journals the nurses kept. One records the process of change as one of 'meeting the unfamiliar, to learning to understand the new practice, to accepting it as a safe way to practise' (Seton 2004, p. 95).

The environment into which these migrant nurses entered was also variable. Some were welcomed, while some were met with degrees of non-acceptance ranging from unhelpfulness to outright racism. While racism is not acceptable in New Zealand, it remains difficult to challenge, particularly where added factors of power, authority, gender and professional status are involved. Most of the nurses accepted adjustment to a new environment as part of the professional adaptation, and worked out ways to learn about their new situations, finding out what they had to do to survive. Some still expressed frustrations, mainly in two fields. Firstly, not using nursing skills, such as venepuncture and suturing, contributed to patient suffering and inefficiency in the nurses' views. It should be noted here that New Zealand nurses do undertake these procedures, but only after formal additional training, and with regular review of skills, as they are 'delegated (from the medical profession) tasks'. Secondly, the migrant nurses were often frustrated by patients exercising their rights to refuse treatment. 'How can you help if that person doesn't want help?', one wondered (Seton 2004, p. 62). The nurses then struggled with finding the balance between allowing that right, educating the patient about the treatment, and how to encourage, promote, or support the treatment without overriding the right to refuse. That they were struggling with this indicates adaptation to a new professional environment.

ADDITIONAL CHALLENGES

A key reason for migration for many nurses is the goal of improving their and their family's economic status. Some nurses are moving from persecution to freedom. When nurses carry with them the duty of providing for their extended family, they may experience a heavy responsibility to gain full registration, get work and begin the process of family re-unification, by which other members of their family may eventually become New Zealand residents. This pressure may make them vulnerable to exploitation both at home and in their new country.

An article published in 2005 outlined how Filipino nurses coming to New Zealand were exploited by unscrupulous agents who charged large fees and then did not provide services (Manchester 2005). Some nurses were charged such large sums that it took one or more years of paying from their wages to make up the debt. Some were bonded for up to three years to small hospitals or rest homes that had paid the agent. A later report (O'Connor 2005) indicated that many similar stories had come to light and outlined the support available to Filipino and other migrant nurses. This second report included a 'happy experience' of another Filipina nurse who outlined how she had checked out the agency she enrolled with, and the constructive support she had received from her New Zealand colleagues.

THE PROFESSIONAL ROLE IN NURSE MIGRATION

The New Zealand Nurses' Organisation (NZNO) takes seriously the professional role of following up on ethical practices in nurse migration issues. Publication of news items, letters, and investigations of the conditions of migrant nurses are part of such actions. New Zealand nurses attend the South Pacific Nurses' Forum, where nurses from Vanuatu, Kiribati, Tonga, Samoa, East Timor, Australia, Tuvalu, Rarotonga, Fiji, Niue, Papua New Guinea and New Zealand gather to share professional nursing issues. The wealthier countries of Australia and New Zealand support their colleagues in smaller nations with funds, knowledge, administrative help, educational opportunities and other resources. For example, in 2002 the NZNO resolved to disseminate research findings to the smaller Pacific Island nations. It was also noted at their conference in 2000 that Fiji nurses were being recruited to New Zealand, and a call was made for greater equity in the recognition of overseas registration in New Zealand. By 2005 the drain of Fiji nurses continued, and the Fiji Nursing Association called on New Zealand to support their claims for improvements in pay and conditions (McIntyre 2005). In 2007, the chief executive of the organisation was again offering support as the military government (post coup) of Fiji attempted to reduce nurses' wages as a means of reducing government expenditure (O'Connor 2007). Thus the NZNO works to support colleagues in other countries to reduce the conditions that force nurses to migrate at the same time as seeking to address the concerns of those who have arrived in New Zealand, as is their legal and moral right.

INTERNATIONAL EXPERIENCES OF MIGRANT NURSES

The experiences of nurses coming to work in New Zealand mirror those of migrant nurses internationally. Migrant nurses report that they are failing to progress (Lipley 2005) and experience racism and exploitation. The question of equity of access for ongoing education for migrant nurses, as well as racial issues, are also recorded (Gerrish & Griffith 2004). Though these reports come from UK experiences, similar stories are found in US experiences with a claim, for Korean nurses, that the initial adjustment phase may last about two to three years, and that an additional five to 10 years are needed to complete adjustment (Yi & Jezewski 2000). (*See also* Chapter 11.)

SUPPORTING MIGRANT NURSES IN NEW ZEALAND

The specific themes of this chapter are the competence and acceptance of migrant nurses. In relation to the global situation, the crisis factors identified by ICN in the position paper *Ethical Nurse Recruitment* remain true (ICN 2001). These principles remain important in 2007. They are, however, organisational and national level principles; what are needed to complement the larger-scale responses are local actions, where individuals put these values into their everyday practice. The five recommendations from Seton's study (2004) relate to successful transition into a professional nursing workforce. Seton suggests a national induction or orientation programme, underpinned by professional development programmes, for people working with migrant nurses. She further recommends the availability of better information for nurses preparing to come to New Zealand. The most important recommendations, however, are those of support for the nurses once they are working in the New Zealand nursing environment. Seton believes that, with appropriate strategies and services, and with common interest groups, transition to professional practice will become more effective and migrant nurses will more quickly feel at home in their new environment.

Seton indicates that it is how individual nurses welcome and support their new colleague that actually makes the difference to how well and how quickly that person becomes an effective member of the health team, and ultimately makes that transition from an alien status to one of becoming a committed citizen in a new country (Seton 2004). What is true for New Zealand nurses is true for a nursing workforce anywhere in the world; for a nurse to recognise an immigrant nurse as a colleague and to support and facilitate that nurse's transition into a new environment is the basis of successful acceptance.

WHAT WOULD BE NEEDED GLOBALLY TO SMOOTH THE TRANSITION TO REGISTERED NURSE PRACTICE IN A NEW COUNTRY FOR IMMIGRANT NURSES?

Increasing similarity among undergraduate programmes leading to registration allows easier comparison and recognition of equivalency. National registration bodies need to be encouraged to set fair assessments, aided by national nursing organisations whose members actually work with the immigrant nurses and must therefore understand the contribution of and the challenges for new colleagues.

The most significant responsibility, once national systems are in place, however, lies with each registered nurse, wherever in the world she or he works with an immigrant nursing colleague. No matter how good or bad the systems, programmes or orientation are, the genuine acceptance of one nurse by another nurse truly signals the universality of nursing.

QUESTIONS FOR DISCUSSION

1 What experiences do you have in relation to working in a new or foreign environment?
2 What experiences do you have of supporting an immigrant nurse and what reflections do you have on what went well or badly, and why?
3 How do you respond when you note unsupportive systems or actions in relation to a new nurse?
4 To what extent do you agree that the duty of care to the new immigrant nurse continues through the registration body all the way to the individual nurse in the workplace?

REFERENCES

ANF. Nurses Reject Random Competency Checks. *Australian Nursing Journal.* 2002; **10**(4): 11.

Cassie F. Workforce Growing: APC stats show. *New Zealand Nursing Review.* 2006; **6**(13): 1.

Clark M. *Workforce Statistics: 2006 update.* Nursing Council of New Zealand's Forum. Auckland: NCNZ; 2006. Available at: http://www.nursingcouncil.org.nz/Workforce%20 Stats.pdf (accessed 17 October 2007).

Farag R. Poor Service From Recruitment Agencies. *Kai Tiaki Nursing New Zealand.* 2006; **12**(2): 3.

Gerrish K, Griffith V. Integration of Overseas Registered Nurses: evaluation of an adaptation programme. *Journal of Advanced Nursing.* 2004; **45**(6): 579–87.

ICN. *Ethical Nurse Recruitment.* 2001. Available at: http://www.icn.ch/psrecruito1.htm (accessed 20 October 2006).

ICN. *Priorities to Address Global Nursing Shortages.* 2006. Available at: http://www.icn.ch/ PR04_06.htm (accessed 29 March 2006).

Lipley N. Call to Meet Individual Needs of Overseas Nurse Recruits. *Nursing Management.* 2005; **12**(6): 5.

Manchester A. Filipino Nurses Suffer Abuse and Exploitation. *Kai Tiaki Nursing New Zealand.* 2005; **11**(4): 12–13.

McIntyre L. Fiji Nurses Prepare for Their Own Pay Campaign. *Kai Tiaki: Nursing New Zealand.* 2005; **11**(3): 12–13.

Mulrooney O. Overseas nurses' registration. (Letter) *Nursing Older People.* 2005; **17**(4): 36.

Nelson S, Purkis ME. Mandatory Reflection: the Canadian reconstitution of the competent nurse. *Nursing Inquiry.* 2004; **11**(4): 247–57.

NMC. *The PREP Handbook.* 2001. Available at: http://www.nmc-uk.org/aDefault.aspx (accessed 16 October 2007).

NMC. *Overseas Nursing Registration.* 2007. Available at: http://www.nmc-uk.org/aArticle. aspx?ArticleID=1653 (accessed 16 October 2007).

O'Connor T. Cultural Safety Training Should be Compulsory. *Kai Tiaki Nursing New Zealand.* 2004; **10**(2): 15.

O'Connor T. Filipino Nurses Glad Their Stories Are Now Public. *Kai Tiaki Nursing New Zealand.* 2005; **11**(6): 14–15.

O'Connor T. Fiji Nurses Ready to Strike Against Government's Austerity measures. *Kai Tiaki Nursing New Zealand.* 2007; **13**(4): 9.

Papps E, Kilpatrick J. Nursing Education in New Zealand: past, present and future. In: Papps E, editor. *Nursing in New Zealand.* Auckland: Pearson Education; 2002. pp. 1–13.

Pearson A. Registration, Regulation and Competence in Nursing. *International Journal of Nursing Practice.* 2005; **11**(5): 191–2.

Reid UV. Regional Examination for Nurse Registation, Commonwealth Caribbean. *International Nursing Review.* 2000; **47**(3): 174–83.

Seton K. Diversity in Action: overseas nurses' perspectives on transition to nursing practice in New Zealand. [Unpublished masters thesis]. Auckland: School of Education, University of Auckland; 2004.

Smolenski MC. Credentialing, Certification, and Competence: issues for new and seasoned nurse practitioners. *Journal of the American Academy of Nurse Practitioners.* 2005; **17**(6): 201–4.

Spoonley P. He Iwi Tahi Tatou? (Are we one people?). *Massey* (Alumnae magazine of Massey University). 2007; **22**(1): 19.

Turton C. Overseas Nurses' Registration. (Letter) *Nursing Older People*. 2005; **17**(4): 36.

Webby T, Barnett J. Caring for Villagers in Vanuatu. *Kai Tiaki Nursing New Zealand*. 2005; **11**(8): 18–20.

Yi M, Jezewski MA. Korean Nurses' Adjustment to Hospitals in the United States of America. *Journal of Advanced Nursing*. 2000; **32**(3): 721–9.

16

Nurses as global citizens: a global health curriculum at the University of Toronto, Canada

Freida S Chavez, Elizabeth Peter and Denise Gastaldo

INTRODUCTION

Globalisation presents nurses with the challenge and ethical responsibility of being competent caregivers for a global community (Leininger 1995; Austin 2004). In order to work in such a context, 'nurses must be able not only to deliver competent care to individuals, but also place individual care within the context of a comprehensive view of complex societies' (Ervin *et al.* 2006). Unfortunately, global health and global citizenship are seldom core components of nursing curricula and, far too frequently, nurses are educated as if they would remain in the same town for the rest of their careers.

Integrating global health as a core component into nursing undergraduate programmes not only increases the competence of nurses to work in a global healthcare economy, but also proves socially and ethically relevant, because nurses should be able to acknowledge their often privileged social positioning as health educators and caregivers to be able to function as global citizens (Lunardi *et al.* 2002; Crigger *et al.* 2006; Nussbaum 1997). We illustrate the possibilities and challenges of undertaking curricular changes to integrate global health at the baccalaureate programme in the Lawrence S Bloomberg Faculty of Nursing, University of Toronto, Canada.

GLOBALISATION AND GLOBAL CITIZENSHIP

Global interdependence calls for all persons across the globe to extend their moral responsibility beyond their local communities and national citizenship and to become citizens of the world (Crigger *et al.* 2006). Martha Nussbaum (1997) describes three capacities necessary for humanity to develop global citizenship. The first is the capacity to examine ourselves and our traditions critically. Reflectivity is needed to question and scrutinise our beliefs, traditions and habits to ensure that they are consistent and justifiable. Nancy Crigger *et al.* (2006) suggest that nursing students need to become sensitised to their own culturally established perspectives on healthcare to become capable of identifying and challenging the underlying values and assumptions of their healthcare system, practice and education.

Nussbaum (1997, p. 10) states that citizens also need 'an ability to see themselves not simply as citizens of some local region or group but also, and above all, as human beings bound to all other human beings by ties of recognition and concern'. Nussbaum's view of global citizenship entails a conception of moral cosmopolitanism, in that all persons are fellow citizens who have equal moral worth and deserve equal moral consideration. Global citizenship, however, does not mean that we need to give up our special and local affections and responsibilities, whether familial, local, national, ethnic or religious. Instead, we need to make all persons part of our community of respect and concern, allowing at times that concern to constrain our local interests.

Narrative imagination is the third capacity. This requires the ability to imagine what it might be like to be a person different from oneself, and to understand the experiences, emotions and desires that another person might have, and to try to comprehend her or his life story. Exposing nurses to other cultures and people is only one aspect of developing this kind of narrative imagination. It also requires a politicised understanding of how others are situated in relationship to oneself and others across the globe. This kind of narrative imagination can best be cultivated by the development of critical thinking skills, which represent an opposition to oppressive power relations along with a commitment to social change, social justice and reflection (Painter 2000).

POSTCOLONIAL FEMINISM

Postcolonialism has emerged in former European colonies living under accentuated social inequities (Loomba 2005). Feminist scholars have explored the multiple intersections of gender and colonial relations, such as women's social locations due to marital status, race, ethnicity or class. Postcolonial feminism emerged as an intellectual and political movement to challenge Western authority to use ethnocentric ideas to explain people's lives in other places and times, celebrating pluralism and critiquing strongly any universalism in knowledge. It uncovers and contests global power relations and cultural hegemony (Rajan & Park 2000). In doing so, it examines how gender, class, race, age, and other social relations and forms of oppression function, and explicates the complex power relations inherent in everyday meanings and realities (Anderson *et al.* 2003).

Using this perspective enables the consideration of multiple voices from distinct social and historical locations when analysing healthcare ideas and practices, rather than privileging Western professionals' views on health (Anderson & McCann 2002). This process should be based on awareness of one's own privileges and assumptions in relation to people in distinct social locations, e.g. otherness constituted by race, gender, class or nationality. This consciousness-raising process should produce and actively search for transformative knowledge and subsequent social action. The strength of this framework is its capacity to shed light on inequities in any global context and to encourage the examination of the complex layered nature of health issues. This approach includes the critique of current global (including Canadian) disparities, such as sexism, racism and the imposition of Eurocentric values over aboriginal Canadian and other indigenous knowledge.

Postcolonial feminism represents an opportunity for undergraduate students to acknowledge their multiple locations as individuals and future professionals. It supports students in challenging certainties as the 'right way' to provide care, and illustrates how all knowledge is the result of power relations in a given place. This framework also points to the need to help students to have experiences of displacement (Bhabha 1994) and to learn lessons from the 'sentence of history' that millions of people around the world experience through living in a diaspora and not belonging to a dominant group. Experiencing being the 'other' while away from home promotes self-knowledge and development. It also sensitises students to the importance of social justice – such as the need to address unjust social institutions and relationships – because from this perspective the experiences of individuals are understood to be embedded within larger political, economic, cultural and social contexts. Internalising a sense of social justice is key to countering the prevailing global trends to privilege market justice as an ethical ideal (Peter 2004).

HEALTH FOR ALL

Global health and nursing should be approached through a balanced view between poverty and communities' resilience and capacity to sustain themselves and to participate in addressing their own pressing needs. The 'enlightened notion of global health as a two-way street allows us all to understand that countries around the world benefit from engaging globally in health, working together to share solutions to shared/common problems' (US Department of Health and Human Services 2006). We recognise that nursing operates within the context of a capitalist world economy wherein the nursing labour force is seen as a commodity (Herdman 2004). There is potential for exploitation and oppression within this environment whose focus has been on economic factors rather than the social and cultural outcomes of globalisation. Any examination of the social determinants of health requires critical appraisal of issues related to social justice, human rights and sustainability on a local and international level (Allen & Ogilvie 2004).

It is important for us as nurses to be aware of the effect that globalisation has on nursing labour markets and fair wages, and to ensure that the internationalisation of nursing education and practice is grounded in a way that 'promotes, sustains and values sociocultural diversity' (Herdman 2004). Marion Allen and Linda Ogilvie (2004) noted that nursing is well positioned to show leadership in the development of curricula that enhance understanding of social inequalities on the local, national and international level and to develop partnerships that are respectful and reciprocal.

In recognition of the link between health, society and globalisation, the need for action to improve health was made explicit by the Bangkok Charter of Health Promotion (2007). From these developments, DeAnne Messias (2001) proposes that a broad framework for global health can be articulated that includes:

a   elimination of poverty and social and economic disparities
b   sustainable and environmentally responsible economic development
c   the creation and introduction of public policies for health
d   the protection of human and reproductive rights
e   the empowerment and rights recognition of women, youth and communities
f   the provision of accessible, affordable and culturally sensitive healthcare services.

Global health can be seen as a new framework to achieve 'Health for All' (WHO 1978).

EDUCATIONAL CONTEXT AND BACKGROUND

In Canada, successful completion of a baccalaureate degree in nursing (BScN), usually a four-year programme, is the minimum educational requirement for entry into practice as a registered nurse. In our faculty, a second-entry or accelerated baccalaureate nursing programme (22 months) runs over the course of two academic years for students who have a previous undergraduate degree or several credits and pre-requisite courses from another discipline. In the second-entry programme, courses are specific to nursing and have the same number of clinical practice hours as those in a four-year baccalaureate programme.

In the context of this programme, we have observed a remarkable interest in international health among students. For instance, for a couple of years students self-organised and raised funds to go abroad in the summer between the first and second year. On return, they shared their experiences. One group presentation described their visit as 'Learning in Paradise'. Faculty members were inspired by the students' interest and intentions, but were concerned by their lack of preparation for a global health practicum, safety issues, as well as the burden they could represent to healthcare professionals hosting them.

FACULTY ENGAGEMENT AND CURRICULA CHANGES

Concomitantly to the students' initiatives, several faculty members centred their work around formulating guiding principles for global health, developing a theoretical framework to ensure that ethical questions regarding colonial thinking in nursing, academic tourism and the risk of students 'practising' on people in need were addressed. An undergraduate international group drafted a proposal, including the identification of global health content in each course and the integration of global health into the curriculum, which was approved by the curriculum committee. From this proposal's outcomes we will focus on two courses described below. The implementation of global health content across the programme is still to be evaluated.

Two concrete outcomes in the process of developing a curriculum conducive to global citizenship were:

a   a new section to be called 'Global Health' in the course Primary Health Care: Nursing Perspectives (NUR 461)

b   a new Global Health Clinical Elective (NUR 480) supported by global placements in Canada and internationally.

CREATION OF A GLOBAL HEALTH SECTION IN PRIMARY HEALTH CARE: NURSING PERSPECTIVES (NUR 461)

The global health section aims at encouraging students to think about health issues from a global perspective, and to move beyond conceptualising health status as an individual or patient issue. It provides a global perspective that helps to examine nursing roles and practices locally and globally. Canadian health issues are linked with global health issues using a primary healthcare 'Health for All' framework. Seminars and discussions integrate primary healthcare principles in relation to major issues, such as nurse migration, social determinants of health, global health inequities, immigrant health and other local and international current issues. Strategies for creating sustainable development and partnerships, capacity building and community empowerment are explored. Case studies and examples of primary healthcare initiatives from both the majority and minority world provide students with a better understanding of primary healthcare internationally. The course content and clinical placements also help students to learn about the local relevance of global health and are closely related to current literature on primary healthcare, global health and the Community Health Nurses of Canada (CHNAC) Standards of Practice.

Currently, we can accommodate only 16 students in this global health section and spaces are taken in the first few hours of registration. Feedback gathered in course evaluation has been very positive, for example:

> Content is very interesting, relevant and useful for my future nursing career. It forces me to reflect on my values and ways of thinking.
>
> The class atmosphere was conducive to open and respectful discussions – great seminar topics.
>
> I really enjoyed the class. I am very inspired and encouraged to become a global health nurse.

CREATION OF A GLOBAL HEALTH CLINICAL ELECTIVE (NUR 480)

After all BScN courses are completed, students have the opportunity to apply for some 15 to 20 places in the Global Health Clinical Elective course. Student interest was very high in the first two years of its existence.

NUR480 provides an opportunity for an enriched, independent experience of clinical practice in resource-constrained settings, both within Canada and internationally. Placements were in primary healthcare clinics in Canadian aboriginal areas and low- and medium-income countries. These places offer an excellent opportunity for the examination of the intersections between health and power, race/ethnicity, gender, social class and nationality. Placements were chosen on the basis of an existing relationship with the University of Toronto, availability of nurse preceptorship and alignment of hosts' needs and students' learning objectives.

In 2006, ten students did four-week placements in Canadian Aboriginal Health in Moose Factory, Ontario; Kep, Cambodia; Addis Ababa, Ethiopia; and Windhoek, Namibia. Placement sites were reviewed for the second year based on student and preceptor feedback, availability of nurse preceptors and language capabilities. A steadfast focus on outcome assessment is important so that faculty can truly assess and critically analyse the value of such placements in a transparent and academically cohesive manner (Bosworth *et al.* 2006).

In 2007, 13 students were placed at Conn River, Newfoundland/Labrador; Oshakati and Windhoek, Namibia; and Karad and Hyderabad, India.

PRE-DEPARTURE PREPARATION

Students worked with faculty members in formulating their learning objectives and preparing for their clinical practice. Judy Mill *et al.* (2005) stress the importance of a pre-departure briefing as well as the benefits of the accompaniment by faculty members. In preparing the students for the clinical placements, we were sensitive to the importance of not further burdening our colleagues in already resource-constrained settings. Needs assessments were conducted so as to ensure that students' duties were in alignment with the specific needs identified by host partners themselves. Seminars emphasised the importance of facilitating partnerships and empowerment in relationships with clients and colleagues. Faculty prepared the students with the following pre-departure seminars.

- Introduction to postcolonial feminist perspective
- Globalisation, social justice and nursing
- Human rights, anti-oppression and nursing
- Cultural competence
- Health and safety abroad programme
- Pre-departure sharing and preparing

APPLYING THE POSTCOLONIAL FEMINIST FRAMEWORK TO GLOBAL HEALTH EXPERIENCE

In order to assist the students to apply the postcolonial framework to their experience, reflective journaling (reflective photo journal recommended) and a reflective evaluation summary were required to identify and explain situations in which their taken-for-granted assumptions have been challenged; they felt discomfort in taking action or felt great confidence in their proposed course of action; they could guide their decisions by a postcolonial approach; they felt like a minority professional/person.

STUDENT EXPERIENCE IN NUR480 PLACEMENTS

Except for Ethiopia, where a faculty member accompanied students, preceptors at the host placement agencies worked with students and were supported by our faculty members through electronic and telephone communication during the placement. Students kept a daily log in order to process events as they occurred and to integrate relevant literature into their reflective journal. This helped them to complete a reflective summary evaluation of their learning opportunities on return, any challenges experienced, and suggestions for strengthening the experience for future students. They also presented such ideas at the information session for prospective students.

Northern Ontario

Two students were placed in the resource-constrained and isolated rural Aboriginal community of Moose Factory in Northern Ontario. This is a very good site to analyse intersections of social class, ethnicity and poverty with health issues. Students worked in the community health centre with nurses and other professionals, and community members. Students reported on issues of poverty, inadequate housing, unemployment, family violence, alcohol and substance abuse, dependence on social assistance and discrimination. Students conducted health educational sessions for a youth summer programme in the community and organised youth educational games and activities, addressing nutrition, diabetes and sexual health. They reported challenges dealing with cultural differences and social and health inequities. They witnessed the importance of traditional healing to the community and the challenge of integrating it in a very Western-centric framework of healthcare.

One student stated in her reflective summary: 'Through my work in Moose Factory, I have learned the various effects of colonization on Aboriginals in Canada. The after-effects of colonization are still extremely apparent in the inequities faced in day-to-day life for Aboriginals in Moose Factory compared to non-Native Canadians.'

Ethiopia

Three students and a faculty member went to Addis Ababa and piloted some teaching sessions as requested by the Amanuel Psychiatric Hospital. The learners included clinical nurses currently enrolled in the Psychiatric Nursing Course at the Amanuel Hospital and senior psychiatric nursing staff. The students' experience involved direct classroom teaching in Addis Ababa and visiting psychiatric nurses in rural health centres. Learning experiences included knowledge and skill development in seminars, didactic teaching, group facilitation, and needs assessment and evaluation. The evaluation indicated that the experience was challenging for undergraduate nurses and would be more suitable for graduate nurses with specialisation in psychiatry/mental health. This feedback was considered and this is now a master's placement.

Consistent with the principle of reciprocal partnerships, two Ethiopian nurse educators came to Toronto for two weeks in September 2006, in order to familiarise themselves with the Canadian context of mental health services and nursing education, and further refinement of the project's next steps.

Cambodia

Three nursing students travelled to Cambodia for four weeks in 2006. Cambodia is one of the poorest countries in Southeast Asia, and there is a continuing struggle to rebuild its social infrastructure, including its healthcare system. Students conducted a community needs assessment in order to gain a better understanding of the health of the Kep community, the organisation of healthcare delivery, and explored potential opportunities for international nursing. They met with villagers, staff and authorities of regional health centres, the Kep Referral Hospital, the Red Cross of Cambodia, a children's orphanage, a primary public school and an HIV village. They also visited the Nursing School in Kampot, the National Maternal and Child Health Center in Phnom Penh, outreach organisations, and conducted a health educational outreach service in a remote village.

One student stated in her reflective summary: 'While it was a very good experience, there were numerous barriers to learning, including language and lack of clinical placements. It was clearly difficult to find clinical placements even for the students who are currently training in Kampot; therefore it would seem that clinical placements would not be the most feasible option for international nursing students in this area. Support on site was good in some placements but not in others.' Based on students' feedback, Cambodia is no longer a clinical site.

Namibia

In 2006, two students went to Windhoek; in 2007, two went to Windhoek and two to Oshakati. They reported on gaining a better understanding of the impact of apartheid. Students learned about the HIV/AIDS pandemic and how it shapes the lives especially of African women and children.

Students worked in a hospital in the community of Katutura, a poverty-stricken area where the spread of HIV/AIDS continues to increase and more children are orphaned each day. They described deplorable living conditions, including complete lack of sanitation and houses made of left-over pieces of sheet metal. Most children living in this neighbourhood did not attend school. Many parents were dying of HIV/AIDS, leaving their children homeless to live in the streets or with their impoverished grandparents. Although apartheid is no longer practised, the poverty caused by the racial segregation has left behind great disparity (Iipinge et al. 2004).

One student quoted in her reflective evaluation: 'On a recent trip to Namibia in sub-Saharan Africa, I had the opportunity to gain a better understanding about the HIV/AIDS pandemic and how it shapes the lives of all men, women and children living in Africa. Coming from a Western background, from a middle-income family, with two university degrees, I am not experienced in the world of suffering of the nature and magnitude I saw in some of the lives of the people I met in Namibia. It is hard to articulate the oppression and discrimination that black women in sub-Saharan Africa face in postcolonial societies from an outsider's perspective.'

EVALUATING THE GLOBAL HEALTH CLINICAL ELECTIVE

The evaluation process has been enhanced for the second year of the course. It now includes oral and written feedback from students, host organisations, and preceptors on site. Evaluation forms have been updated, with a more rigorous student clinical evaluation component completed by both students and site and faculty preceptors. After three years of implementation, we plan to do a systematic evaluation of this course, taking into account barriers and facilitators for teaching and learning global citizenship, both within the faculty curriculum and the different placements offered.

FINAL REMARKS AND FUTURE DIRECTIONS

In 1978, the UN stated that by the year 2000 health would be a possibility for all human beings (WHO 1978). Since the early 1990s some nursing academics and practitioners have been calling on nursing organisations and institutions to open classroom doors for theory and practice regarding global issues, and yet in 2007 undergraduate nursing education has neither led nor imparted the fundamentals of a global health curriculum; the current curriculum is mainly reactionary rather than a proactive force in shaping the future of the profession and healthcare systems (Mill *et al.* 2005; Ervin *et al.* 2006).

Global health as a core element of the nursing undergraduate curriculum in preparing nurses to be competent caregivers, educators, and global citizens committed to an agenda of health for all, is relevant. Our evolving process, as we integrate global health in the curriculum, is one approach, hopefully providing insights for other faculties on similar journeys.

We have learned that the education of nurses as global citizens requires a transformative pedagogical agenda for both lecturers and students. Those teaching global health have to articulate principles coherently, such as the well-known 'Health for All'. Pedagogical practices in class and during preceptorship need to be geared towards recognising that all knowledge is contextual; Western scientific knowledge is produced in market-oriented societies; sustainable partnerships depend on respect for a myriad of positions on the same topic; social justice should be the criterion for negotiation.

Students may already be on the path of building their own global citizenship from previous educational opportunities. However, in nursing they have to overcome the dominant emphasis on individual care, commonly disconnected from social, economic and cultural contexts, and engage with critical thinking and reflection, developing the capacity of identifying tensions between one's own professional interests, local and global interests.

Nurses who can exercise their global citizenship professionally should work from these premises:

❑ that people's experiences of health and illness are culturally and geographically located, with the majority of the world living under severe social and economic inequities

❑ that global health nurses should have the ability to address the health concerns of the majority of the world's population

❑ that nursing labour has become a market commodity

❑ that projects related to 'Health for All' engage in the construction of sustainable, publicly run sanitation and safe water programmes, affordable, healthy food and housing initiatives, building on national healthcare systems.

QUESTIONS FOR DISCUSSION

1 How can global health in nursing education be integrated when most lecturers and professors have not been educated in the subject and many conservative thinkers among us would claim that a global 'Health for All' social justice framework is a personal or political choice beyond the scope of practice?

2 How can social transformation among nurses be addressed when there is a strong belief of powerlessness in the profession and, therefore, nurses do not perceive themselves as agents of change and as capable of transforming healthcare or political structures?

REFERENCES

Allen M, Ogilvie L. Internationalization of Higher Education: potential and pitfalls for nursing education. *International Nursing Review*. 2004; **51**: 73–80.

Anderson J, McCann K. Toward a Post-colonial Feminist Methodology in Nursing Research: exploring the convergence of post-colonial and black feminist scholarship. *Nursing Research* 2002; **9**(3): 7–27.

Anderson J, Perry J, Blue C, *et al.* 'Rewriting' Cultural Safety Within the Postcolonial and Postnational Feminist Project: toward new epistemologies of healing. *Advances in Nursing Science*. 2003; **26**(3): 196–214.

Austin W. Global Health Challenges, Human Rights, and Nursing Ethics. In: Storch J, Rodney P, Starzomski R, editors. *Toward a Moral Horizon: nursing ethics in leadership and practice*. Don Mills, ON: Pearson Education Canada; 2004. pp. 339–56.

Bangkok Charter for Health Promotion in a Globalized World. 2007. Available at: http://www.who.int/healthpromotion/conferences/6gchp/bangkok_charter/en/index.html (accessed 26 September 2007).

Bhabha H. *The Location of Culture*. London: Routledge; 1994.

Bosworth TL, Haloburdo EP, Hetrick C, *et al.* International Partnerships to Promote Quality

Care: faculty groundwork, student projects, and outcomes. *Journal of Continuing Education in Nursing.* 2006; **37**(1): 32–8.

Crigger N, Brannigan M, Baird M. Compassionate Nursing Professionals as Good Citizens of the World. *Advances in Nursing Science.* 2006; **29**(4): 15–26.

Ervin NE, Bickes JT, Schim SM. Environments of Care: a curriculum model for preparing a new generation of nurses. *Journal of Nursing Education.* 2006; **45**(2): 75–80.

Herdman E. Globalization, Internationalization and Nursing. *Nursing and Health Sciences.* 2004; **6**: 237–8.

Iipinge SN, Hofnie K, Freidman S. *The Relationship Between Gender Roles and HIV Infection in Namibia.* Windhoek, Namibia: University of Namibia Press; 2004.

Leininger M. *Transcultural Nursing: concepts, theories, research and practices.* 2nd ed. New York: McGraw-Hill; 1995.

Loomba A. *Colonialism/Postcolonialism.* 2nd ed. London: Routledge; 2005.

Lunardi V, Peter E, Gastaldo D. Are Submissive Nurses Ethical?: reflecting on power anorexia. *Revista Brasileira de Enfermagem.* 2002; **55**(2): 183–8.

Messias DK. Globalization, Nursing and Health for All. *Journal of Nursing Scholarship.* 2001; **33**(1): 9–15.

Mill JE, Yonge OJ, Cameron BS. Challenges and Opportunities of International Clinical Practice. *International Journal of Nursing Education Scholarship.* 2005; **2**(1): 1–13.

Nussbaum MC. *Cultivating Humanity: a classical defense of reform in liberal education.* Cambridge & London: Harvard University Press; 1997.

Painter J. Critical Human Geography. In: Johnston RJ, Gregory D, Pratt G, Watts M, editors. *The Dictionary of Human Geography.* 4th ed. Oxford: Blackwell Publishers; 2000. pp. 126–8.

Peter E. Home Health Care and Ethics. In: Storch J, Rodney P, Starzomski R, editors. *Toward a Moral Horizon: nursing ethics in leadership and practice.* Don Mills, ON: Pearson Education Canada; 2004. pp. 248–61.

Rajan RS, Park Y. Postcolonial Feminism/Postcolonial and Feminism. In: Schwarz H, Ray S, editors. *A Companion for Postcolonial Studies.* Oxford: Blackwell; 2000. pp. 53–71.

US Department of Health and Human Services. *Frequently Asked Questions.* Available at: http://www.globalhealth.gov/faq.shtm (accessed 10 April 2006).

WHO. *Declaration of Alma Ata.* New York: WHO; 1978. Available at: http://www.who.int/hpr/NPH/docs/declaration_almaata.pdf (accessed 4 May 2008).

SECTION 6

Patient safety

17

Globalisation and pandemic: fighting against the spread of infectious diseases

Huey-Ming Tzeng and Chang-Yi Yin

INTRODUCTION

From a global perspective of healthcare in relation to infectious diseases, there are two possible ways forward: 'merging' or 'homogenisation'. Merging considers that all nations are an organic whole, where public health resources are owned and controlled primarily by the well-developed nations. These resources can be allocated to the less-developed nations at the discretion of well-developed nations. Homogenisation means that all nations reach the same level and balance in their development, production, supply and demand; public health resources are shared to achieve the overall global health (Yin 2003).

Should globalisation therefore aim to merge all nations into an organic whole or should it have nations become homogenised and balanced in every way? Most definitions of globalisation have focused on the economic implications of the increased integration of economic markets. Some have captured the interplay of the economic, political, cultural and social dimensions of globalisation (Axfor 2000). In these, the purpose of globalisation has been primarily to achieve the *merging* of markets.

In contrast, at the Millennium Summit in 2000 at the UN, the agenda to advance global health in the twenty-first century included eight development goals:

1   eradicate extreme poverty and hunger
2   achieve universal primary education
3   promote gender equality and empower women
4   reduce child mortality
5   improve maternal health

6 combat HIV/AIDS, malaria and other diseases
7 ensure environmental sustainability
8 develop a global partnership for development (UN 2000).

This agenda promoted the *homogenisation* aim of globalization.

In this chapter we address the questions: is globalisation leading to merging or homogenisation? Has globalisation contributed to the spread of human-to-human infectious diseases? What should nurses, working across the continuum of healthcare, know about globalisation? By reading this chapter, nurses may gain a macro-perspective of healthcare in the current movement to globalisation.

MERGING IS ONE OF THE CONTRIBUTORS TO THE GLOBAL THREAT OF INFECTIOUS DISEASES

Networking activities, including international travel and trade, are constantly increasing, promoting the concept of the 'global village'. Along with positive effects of such globalisation, this can lead to increasing exposures to disease-causing agents formerly confined to small, remote areas. Globalisation has made the spread of infectious diseases to distant places more possible then ever, most likely from countries that are considered to have a low or medium level of human development to countries with a high level of human development. The UN Development Programme (2006) has set indications for measuring high, medium, or low human development (*see* Table 17.1).

Examples of recent emerging or re-emerging infectious diseases of global concern include SARS, HIV, a new form of cholera, haemolytic uraemic syndrome, hepatitis C, legionnaires' disease, Lyme disease, tuberculosis, and most recently avian (H5N1) influenza. Possible contributors to the emergence and re-emergence of infectious diseases are linked to rapid and intense international travel, increased exposure of people to disease vectors and reservoirs in nature, and overcrowding in cities with poor sanitation (WHO 1997).

HUMAN DEVELOPMENT CLASSIFICATIONS WITH RESPECT TO THE SARS AND H5N1 EPIDEMICS

We used SARS and H5N1 avian flu as examples to illustrate the epidemiological trends of the spread of newly emerging infectious diseases. The statistics in the UN *Human Development Report 2005* and two summary reports provided by the WHO were combined, as shown in Tables 17.1 and 17.2 (UN Development Programme 2006; WHO 2007a, 2007b, 2007c). These two tables include the following information: (1) a summary of probable SARS cases with onset of

TABLE 17.1 Human development classifications of the areas with probable SARS cases with onset of illness from 1 November 2002 to 31 July 2003 (United Nations Development Programme 2006, World Health Organization 2007a, 2007b)

Country*	HDI[1]	HDC[2]	Cumulative Cases/Deaths	Date onset first probable case	Local transmission[3]
China	0.755	Medium	5327/349	16–Nov–2002	N/A
China, Hong Kong	0.916	High	1755/299	15–Feb–2003	Yes
Canada	0.949	High	251/43	23–Feb–2003	Yes
Viet Nam	0.704	Medium	63/5	23–Feb–2003	Yes
Singapore	0.907	High	238/33	24–Feb–2003	Yes
United States	0.944	High	27/0	24–Feb–2003	N/A
China, Taiwan	N/A	N/A	346/37	25–Feb–2003	N/A
Philippines	0.758	Medium	14/2	25–Feb–2003	N/A
Australia	0.955	High	6/0	26–Feb–2003	N/A
Republic of Ireland	0.946	High	1/0	27–Feb–2003	N/A
United Kingdom	0.939	High	4/0	1–Mar–2003	N/A
Germany	0.930	High	9/0	9–Mar–2003	None
Switzerland	0.947	High	1/0	9–Mar–2003	N/A
Thailand	0.778	Medium	9/2	11–Mar–2003	None
Italy	0.934	High	4/0	12–Mar–2003	N/A
Malaysia	0.796	Medium	5/2	14–Mar–2003	N/A
Romania	0.792	Medium	1/0	19–Mar–2003	N/A
France	0.938	High	7/1	21–Mar–2003	N/A
Spain	0.928	High	1/0	26–Mar–2003	N/A
Sweden	0.949	High	5/0	28–Mar–2003	N/A
Mongolia	0.679	Medium	9/0	31–Mar–2003	N/A
South Africa	0.658	Medium	1/1	3–Apr–2003	N/A
Indonesia	0.697	Medium	2/0	6–Apr–2003	N/A
Kuwait	0.844	High	1/0	9–Apr–2003	N/A
New Zealand	0.933	High	1/0	20–Apr–2003	N/A
India	0.602	Medium	3/0	25–Apr–2003	N/A
Republic of Korea	0.901	High	3/0	25–Apr–2003	N/A
Russian Federation	0.795	Medium	1/0	5–May–2003	N/A
China, Macao	N/A	N/A	1/0	5–May–2003	N/A
Total			**8096/774**		

Notes:

* Data is sorted by the date of onset of the first probable case.

(Notes continued overleaf.)

1 HDI (Human Development Index). HDI is a composite index that measures the average achievements in a country in three dimensions of human development: (1) life expectancy at birth (reflecting a long and healthy life), (2) the adult literacy rate and the combined gross enrolment ratio for primary, secondary, and tertiary schools (measuring knowledge), and (3) GDP per capita in purchasing power parity U.S. dollars (as an indicator of a decent standard of living). The HDI in the *Human Development Report 2005* refers to the world environment in 2003, including 175 member countries of the United Nations, Hong Kong, China, and the Occupied Palestinian Territories (United Nations Development Programme 2006).

2 HDC (Human Development Classifications). Countries were classified into three clusters: (1) high human development (with an HDI of 0.800 or above), (2) medium human development (0.500–.0799), and (3) low human development (less than 0.500) (United Nations Development Programme 2006).

3 Local transmission was determined based on the data of cumulative number of reported suspect and probable cases (SARS) from 1 February 2003 to 17 March 2003. If imported cases were immediately isolated, these areas were not considered as affected areas (World Health Organization 2007b).

N/A: Not available.

TABLE 17.2 Human development classifications of the areas with confirmed human cases of avian influenza A (H5N1) reported to the World Health Organization (as of 29 January 2007) (United Nations Development Programme 2006, World Health Organization 2007c)

Country*	HDI[1]	HDC[2]	No. of cases and deaths (cases/deaths) by country by year					
			2003	2004	2005	2006	2007	Total
Viet Nam	0.704	Medium	3/3	29/20	61/19	0/0	0/0	93/42
Indonesia	0.697	Medium	0/0	0/0	19/12	56/46	6/5	81/63
Thailand	0.778	Medium	0/0	17/12	5/2	3/3	0/0	25/17
China	0.755	Medium	1/1	0/0	8/5	13/8	0/0	22/14
Egypt	0.659	Medium	0/0	0/0	0/0	18/10	1/1	19/11
Turkey	0.750	Medium	0/0	0/0	0/0	12/4	0/0	12/4
Azerbaijan	0.729	Medium	0/0	0/0	0/0	8/5	0/0	8/5
Cambodia	0.571	Medium	0/0	0/0	4/4	2/2	0/0	6/6
Iraq	N/A	N/A	0/0	0/0	0/0	3/2	0/0	3/2
Djibouti	0.495	Low	0/0	0/0	0/0	1/0	0/0	1/0
Total			4/4	46/32	97/42	116/80	7/6	270/164

Notes:

* Data is sorted by the number of cases (from high to low).

1 and 2: *See* the notes of **Table 1**.

N/A: Not available.

illness from 1 November 2002 to 31 July 2003, and (2) the cumulative number of confirmed human cases of avian influenza A (H5N1) reported to WHO.

As shown in Table 17.1, SARS originated in the People's Republic of China, where it was first reported on 16 November 2002, and then spread to 28 other countries, including 16 with either high or medium levels of human development. Table 17.2 indicates that most probably because of poor public health conditions, all ten countries with confirmed human cases of H5N1 avian influenza reported to WHO were countries with a medium level of human development. Pathogens do not recognise national boundaries or if a country is industrialised. The next country to have a confirmed human case of H5N1 avian influenza could be a country with high, medium or low development.

HOMOGENISATION IS NEEDED

Is homogenisation the solution to prevent global threats of new or re-emerging infectious diseases? Routine surveillance of infectious disease outbreaks is no longer relevant for local areas only and is not limited to national-level public health programmes. Outbreaks require regional and global alerts and response mechanisms to ensure rapid access to technical advice and resources, as well as to support national public health capacity. For the same reason, in April 2000 the WHO (2007d) established the Global Outbreak Alert and Response Network; these regulations are binding across all nations.

The development of international health organisations and regulations for dealing with the threat of infectious diseases should be developed and implemented as soon as possible (Stern & Markel 2004). However, such a global strategy would be successful only if such efforts aim to promote a homogenised and balanced global development, production, supply and demand across all countries, regardless of high, medium or low human development (UN Development Programme 2006; Yin 2003).

Rather than taking on the role of fire fighters when an outbreak occurs, the more highly developed countries should provide the financial and personnel support for the education, medical and public health systems of those countries that are less developed, in order to avert more effectively the threat of infectious diseases from being transmitted to other parts of the world. The more highly developed countries should therefore be proactive, rather than reactive. In addition, to address the threat of infectious diseases appropriately, medical personnel from developing countries also require continuous training and access to sufficient infection control measures and equipment.

IMPLICATIONS FOR NURSING PRACTICE

Challenges to provide holistic patient care

Because of immigration and constant travel across continents for business and leisure for people from various settings, the patients in any medical system are highly diverse. Patient care therefore has become increasingly complex. The trend towards globalisation is creating challenges for nurses to provide holistic patient care, including having to deal with unfamiliar infectious diseases and the taboos of patients and their families, often related to their religions and traditional values.

Nurses' cultural and transnational competencies, e.g. patient-focused interpersonal skills, need to be relevant and considered as one of the ethical demands of the globalisation process of nursing. The purpose of being equipped with cultural and transnational competencies is to be prepared for ethnically and socially differing clinical encounters at the interface of religion and culture-appropriate care (Koehn 2006).

Nurses are at the front lines

Nurses are at the front lines because they have most contact with patients. Their fears concerning new or re-emerging infectious diseases should be considered before the emergence of a pandemic. It is critical that nurses do not themselves become part of a panicking public. For clinical nurses, being healthy, continually acquiring updated information on caring for any patients who may have a new or re-emerging infectious disease, and observing the required standards for infection control precautions, are essential (Tzeng and Yin 2006a, 2006b).

Political duty

Nurses have a duty to sustain nursing care quality and patient safety, as well as clinical practice, by demanding the right and sufficient tools for infection control measures. The equipment, e.g. masks, gowns, and so on, to fight infectious diseases must be supplied by their governments, otherwise nurses cannot be effective practitioners, and risk becoming infected themselves.

Intentionally or unintentionally, this issue is perhaps often overlooked by nurses, governments and the public. Governments everywhere are saving money, and therefore might want to be concerned about finance more than detailed care. When a government can spare a lump sum on promoting public health, e.g. prevention of the spread of SARS and tuberculosis, such monies should be spent in the right places. Nurses have the political duty to ensure that they get what they need for quality patient care from their work institutions and through their government agencies.

What nurses can do to be politically active for themselves and their associations is to participate in supervising governments; for example, on spending money and resources on promoting the health of the public and preventing occupational hazards in nurses' working places. It is also important to lobby legislators for making new or changing policies related to patient safety and having a safe work environment for nurses. Nurses must also learn how to use the mass media, e.g. television, newspapers and websites, to illustrate their perspectives, and to obtain consensus among nurses locally as well as in international forums.

Learning about patient care experiences from one another

The trend seems always to be that nurses working in the low-income or medium or low human development countries, i.e. those countries with less human resources in medical staff and less advanced medical technology, have to learn from high-income or high human development countries. It has increasingly to be accepted that high-income countries must learn from the practice of the low-income countries, otherwise the concept of the 'global village' is simply that of a dictatorship. For example, early in the 2003 SARS epidemic, the WHO experts and other medical professionals and scientists from highly developed countries learned about the experience of caring for the SARS patients in China, Viet Nam and Taiwan. Medical and nursing experts there had collected information related to treatment and effective infection control measures of SARS and communicated these via on-site visits, professional journals and documentation, video conferencing, the Internet, and so on. This is a recent example of high-income countries learning from the practice of low-income countries in dealing with global health issues, and will no doubt be repeated increasingly.

Skill migration of nurses is another concern

Skill migration of nurses has also been perceived as a concern. Because of a serious shortage of nurses in industrialised countries, nurses with professional training may choose to immigrate to a high human development country to receive better pay and an improved working environment. Consequently, the overall medical care and public health services of the medium or low human development countries that export qualified and skilled nurses to more highly developed countries suffer.

The roles played by nurses and nursing leaders in globalisation

Nursing leaders and educators can actively promote and increase the knowledge of nurses who are working in medium or low human development countries about newly emerging infectious diseases. Such efforts demand funding from the UN and local governments. Nursing scholars and educators in countries with different levels of human development should collaborate to offer advanced nursing courses about the healthcare issues related to fighting against the spread of emerging infectious diseases. Utilising advanced web-based teaching sessions may reach more nurses in every part of the world.

CONCLUSION

New or re-emerging diseases cause human suffering and create a high economic burden, as well as the potential for spreading internationally. Nursing and other caring disciplines must work together to combat emerging infectious diseases of global concern (Lashley 2004). To improve global health, and in order to attain all the Millennium Development Goals, it is important to push highly developed countries to become actively involved in the homogenisation efforts of globalisation. Balancing the consequences and merging all nations into an organic whole is necessary to increase the integration of economic markets (Yin 2003).

REFERENCES

Axfor B. 2000. Globalization. In: Browning G, Halcli A, Webster F, editors. *Understanding Contemporary Society: theories of the present*. London: SAGE; 2000. pp. 238–51.

Koehn PH. Globalization, Migration Health, and Educational Preparation for Transnational Medical Encounters. *Global Health*. 2006; **2**(1): 2.

Lashley FR. Emerging Infectious Diseases: vulnerabilities, contributing factors and approaches. *Expert Review of Anti-infective Therapy*. 2004; **2**(2): 299–316.

Stern AM, Markel H. International Efforts to Control Infectious Diseases, 1851 to the Present. *Journal of the American Medical Association*. 2004; **292**(12): 1474–9.

Tzeng HM, Yin CY. Is H5N1 Like a Ghost-flu That Can Cause a Pandemic in Humans? *Nursing Ethics*. 2006a; **13**: 219–21.

Tzeng HM, Yin CY. Nurses' Professional Obligations and Their Fears of Facing a Possible Human-to-human Avian Influenza Pandemic. *Nursing Ethics*. 2006b **13**: 455–70.

UN Development Programme. *Human Development Report 2005 (Appendix: Human development indicators*, pp. 209–328). 2006. Available at: http://hdr.undp.org/reports/global/2005/ (accessed 1 February 2007).

UN. *United Nations Millennium Declaration: Resolution adopted by the General Assembly (54/281- Organization of the Millennium Summit of the United Nations, 18 September 2000*). Available at: http://www.un.org/millennium/ (accessed 1 February 2007).

WHO. *World Health Day, 7 April 1997: Emerging infectious diseases*. 1997. Available from: http://www.who.int/docstore/world-health-day/en/whday1997.html (accessed 1 February 2007).

WHO. *Summary of Probable SARS Cases with Onset of Illness from 1 November 2002 to 31 July 2003*. 2007a. Available at: http://www.who.int/csr/sars/country/table2004_04_21/en/ print.html (accessed 1 February 2007).

WHO. *Cumulative Number of Reported Suspect and Probable Cases (SARS): 1 February 2003 to*

17 March 2003. 2007b. Available from: http://www.who.int/csr/sars/country/table/en/index.html (accessed 1 February 2007).

WHO. *Cumulative Number of Confirmed Human Cases of Avian Influenza A/(H5N1) Reported to WHO, 29 January 2007*. 2007c. Available at: http://www.who.int/csr/disease/avian_influnza/country/cases_table_2007_01_29/en/index.html (accessed 1 February 2007).

WHO. *Epidemic and Pandemic Alert and Response (EPR): global outbreak alert and response network.* 2007d. Available at: http://www.who.int/csr/outbreaknetwork/en/ (accessed 1 February 2007).

Yin CY. The History of the Development of Globalization and the Crisis of Promoting Localization in Taiwan (in Mandarin). *New Scope in Society (Taiwan)*. 2003; **5**: 4–12.

18

International recruitment of nurses and patient safety: an ethical dilemma of individual rights and distributive justice

Sylvia Bertram

INTRODUCTION

This chapter will explore the worldwide shortage of registered nurses, its linkage to patient safety, international recruitment of nurses, and the ethical dilemmas it creates. I will begin with a definition of globalisation and a brief review of the global shortage of registered nurses related to patient safety, then consider international recruitment of nurses, discuss autonomy and distributive justice, and conclude with an ethical dilemma case study with questions for consideration.

GLOBALISATION, SHORTAGE OF REGISTERED NURSES AND PATIENT SAFETY

Globalisation refers to world systems that are distinct from national ones; these systems involve the transfer of economic, political and socio-cultural values across borders, potentially blurring national boundaries (Herdman 2004). How globalisation affects a country is dependent on its economy, history, culture, tradition and priorities. The provision of healthcare to citizens of each country can be influenced by globalisation, depending on its own national systems. Since nurses comprise the largest group of healthcare providers (Buerhaus *et al.* 2000) and are an integral part of a national health system, when a shortage exists, its impact can be felt nationally.

A nursing shortage is an imbalance between nursing skill requirements (number of nurses) and the actual availability of nurses. However, 'a nursing shortage is not just an organizational challenge or a topic for economic analysis; it has a major negative impact on healthcare. Failure to deal with a nursing shortage

– be it local, regional, national or global – is likely to lead to failure to maintain or improve health care' (Buchan & Calman 2005, p. 11). Globally, the number of nurses available to care for patients does not meet the ever-increasing demand for the services they provide. For example, the US Department of Health and Human Service's National Center for Health Workforce Analysis noted that the US had a shortfall of 110 707 nurses in 2000 and predicts a shortfall of 275 215 in 2010 and 808 416 in 2020 (US Bureau of Health Professions 2000).

WHO measures shortages with nurse-to-people ratios that can vary from region to region within a country, country to country and continent to continent. In the US, the Health Resources and Services Administration (HRSA) reports that the average ratio of nurses was 858 per 100 000 people in 2005 (HRSA 2005) as compared with Ethiopia which had 21 nurses per 100 000 people (WHO 2006). The average ratio in Europe is similar to that in the US, with 847 nurses per 100 000 people in the UK (WHO 2006). The average nurse-to-population ratio in high-income countries is almost eight times greater than in low-income countries. Low availability of nurses in many developing countries is exacerbated by geographical maldistribution; there are even fewer nurses available in rural and remote areas. Factors contributing to the nursing shortage vary in different parts of the world.

In the US, multiple factors contributing to the increasing registered nurse shortage include a growing population, the demographic double problem of an ageing workforce caring for an increasingly older population, trying to replace nurses retiring in the next ten years, and coping with a reduction in people interested in entering nursing (Buchan 2002). One example of a variation within a country is afforded by the state of California in the US. While the average nurse-to-population ratio in the US was 858 nurses per 100 000 people in 2005, California had a rate of 590 per 100 000 people (HRSA 2005). Other areas of the world have different contributing factors to the nursing shortage.

In sub-Saharan Africa, contributing factors to the nursing shortage include meagre pay, inadequate sanitation that puts the nurses' own health at risk, shortage of basic supplies, and a high incidence of diseases such as HIV/AIDS that cost the lives of many patients and nurses.

The current global shortage of nurses represents a serious threat to patient safety and quality of healthcare (ICN 2001). The Institute of Medicine defines patient safety as the freedom from accidental injury due to medical care, or medical errors (Kohn *et al.* 1999). The National Patient Safety Foundation (2000) identified three defining characteristics of patient safety: prevention and amelioration of adverse outcomes related to healthcare, the interaction of all elements within a healthcare organisation's systems, and patient safety as a subset of quality of care. Nurses are the key source of patient care.

Hospitals in most countries lack adequate staff to provide care to their patients. Evidence links adequate numbers of nurses to positive healthcare outcomes (Needleman & Buerhaus 2003). Adequate numbers of nurses to provide care are a critical element to patient health and safety. Individuals responsible for providing healthcare, whether at the local, community, state or national level, have a moral obligation to do everything possible to ensure that healthcare is provided to their constituency. Since many countries do not have enough nurses to provide needed healthcare, they resort to recruitment of nurses from other countries to meet their needs. The economic challenges presented by a shortage of nurses in developing countries take precedence over the individual nurses' needs.

INTERNATIONAL RECRUITMENT OF NURSES

International recruitment of nurses has intensified with the global shortage of nurses and is discussed widely in the literature. Debates range from multiple factors contributing to the nursing shortage, to references to developed countries as manipulative in their recruitment practices as they poach nurses from developing countries, leaving those countries to suffer with inadequate numbers of nurses to provide necessary healthcare. The ethical nature of international recruitment is also being questioned.

Migration of nurses from one country to another is a longstanding practice and is considered common (Seloilwe 2005). For years the migration of nurses was from developed countries to developing countries. The trend now is for nurses from developing countries to migrate to developed countries (Seloilwe 2005; Carney 2005; Singh *et al.* 2003).

The migration of foreign nurses has positive aspects as well as challenges and opportunities. Positive aspects of migration for countries include an increase in culturally diverse nurses to provide care to a culturally diverse population, increased numbers of nurses to provide care to patients and for many nurses, an improved quality of life for themselves and their family. Opportunities for individual nurses are many and include the lure of developed countries with higher salaries, the ability to support families at home, enhanced career opportunities, and improved working and living conditions (Xu & Zhang 2005). It has also been said that the international migration of nurses possesses the potential for being a mechanism of empowerment for nurses from developing countries (Meleis 2003).

Not all countries view the migration of their nurses to developed countries as a loss. Historically, the Philippines has educated more nurses than it needs, exporting the nurses to work in other countries so that they can send money home. This situation seems to be changing as the continued migration has left shortages of nurses to provide care in the Philippines (Buchan & Sochalski 2004). India and China, with some limitations related to specific areas or states within each country, currently experience unemployment and underemployment of nurses in their respective countries. Advertising for Indian nurses available to migrate to developed countries abounds.

There is no quick fix to the global nursing shortage, and developed countries have an advantage in the ability to recruit nurses from developing countries that developing countries do not have. When a developing country has a serious shortage of nurses and some nurses opt to emigrate, they leave behind a more stressful work environment and a reduced standard of care, leading to diminished patient safety (Aiken *et al.* 2002; Needleman *et al.* 2002).

Is it unfair that developing countries, which cannot offer what richer developed countries can in salary, benefits, and living conditions, lose their nurses? Is it cheaper to take from another country than to train nurses? Do developing countries save money at the expense of the poor? These are moral issues and beg the question: is international recruiting of nurses an ethical practice?

THE ETHICS OF INTERNATIONAL RECRUITMENT OF NURSES

The steady increase in international recruitment of nurses has lead to the creation of standards to guide the recruiting practice. Countries such as the UK (DH 1999; DH 2004) and the US (American Public Health Association 2005) have issued international recruitment guidelines. In general, the guidelines prohibit recruiting from countries experiencing nurse shortages unless there is an explicit government-to-government agreement to promote recruitment. One exception to the guidelines is the unsolicited application of international nurses. In 2001, the ICN issued the position statement *Ethical Nurse Recruitment*, focusing on the fundamental rights of individual nurses to move wherever they choose (ICN 2001). When comparing the guidelines issued by a country with those of a professional organisation, there is a difference in focus between the interests of the country versus those of individual nurses, and this can create an ethical dilemma (Xu & Zhang 2005).

AUTONOMY AND DISTRIBUTIVE JUSTICE

An ethical dilemma is created when a conflict appears between moral imperatives, in which to obey one would result in transgressing another. Often it is a choice between two nearly evenly balanced alternatives, or between two moral principles or rules in a given situation (Beauchamp & Childress 2001).

In order to enhance ethical dialogue and facilitate ethical decision making, it is essential to select consciously a theoretical framework on which to base discussion. The framework chosen for ethical decision making here is that of principlism (Beauchamp & Childress 2001). Principlism posits that widely held principles provide a starting point for moral judgement and provide guidelines for ethical dilemmas. The two principles selected for the ethical dilemma regarding international recruiting of nurses during a time of shortage are autonomy and distributive justice.

The principle of autonomy – the right of individual nurses to freedom of choice – is juxtaposed with the principle of distributive justice, which speaks to the fair distribution of resources for the common good in a given country. Taking desperately needed nurses from poorer countries appears to be unjust. Restricting nurses from leaving a poor country denies individual freedom of choice. An autonomous action takes into account a person's ability to act intentionally, with reasonable understanding and reasonable absence of controlling influences (Beauchamp & Childress 2001).

The principle of distributive justice refers to equitable, fair and appropriate allocation of goods or services determined by justified norms from cooperative agreements within a society. Problems arise with distributive justice when there is scarcity or a limited supply relative to demand (Beauchamp & Childress 2001).

All countries need to meet the healthcare needs of their population; this is the principle of distributive justice. Is it therefore ethical for developed countries to recruit nurses from less-developed (in terms of money as well as number of nurses to care for the population) countries? Does it depend on the resources within the country hiring nurses? What role does the exporting of nurses play in the economic well-being of the people of the donor country? Are the families of the exported nurses better off financially? Does the decrease in nurses providing care endanger the health and safety of the sending country's citizens?

ETHICAL DILEMMA CASE STUDY

The global shortage of nurses and the resulting international recruitment of nurses has ethical dilemmas for nurses as well as for countries. The questions asked here can provide an opportunity for dialogue with others or for individual introspection regarding a potential resolution to this ethical dilemma. Some readers may be satisfied with the answers while others may not be content with the resolution. This is by no means a comprehensive dialogue regarding an ethical dilemma and intends mainly to provide some questions to consider in the search for a tolerable answer.

Ayanna is from a small town in the eastern Amhara Regional State of Ethiopia. She attended nursing school in Addis Ababa, the capital of Ethiopia, and speaks fluent English. She is a 30-year-old widow and the primary financial support for her ageing parents; she has six years of hospital experience in a very poor small-town hospital. Ethiopia has a severe shortage of nurses and unsafe working conditions. She was actively recruited by a hospital in the US and has a contract to work in place.

Questions for consideration

1 **Define the dilemma**

The dilemma can be defined using several different approaches. A first approach is through primacy of interests, a second addresses the rights of an individual versus a group, and a third might be through addressing an obligation to self versus duty. The primacy of interests looks at the interest of one party over another; in this case the interests of the country versus a nurse's individual interests. Ethiopia is interested in having an adequate supply of nurses to provide healthcare to its citizens, while Ayanna is interested in a safe working environment and being able to care financially for her parents. The second approach to defining a dilemma is addressing the right of an individual nurse's self-determination versus the rights of citizens to have access to healthcare provided by nurses. A third possible approach is to address the obligation of a nurse to her or his family versus the obligation to duty providing healthcare to the citizens of a country. What approach influences your thinking most?

2 **What values are at stake in the dilemma?**

Potential values at stake include an individual's right to make choices, access to healthcare for a country's citizens, and enough nurses to provide care.

3 **What principles are at stake in this dilemma?**

In this case, the principles have already been chosen. The principles are respect for autonomy of the individual versus distributive justice, meeting the healthcare needs and safety of the citizens of Ethiopia, including the health and safety of Ayanna herself.

Other potential questions are:

4 **Autonomy**

❑ Does Ayanna have the right to choose where she lives and works?

❑ Who is Ayanna responsible to and for?

❑ Does Ayanna herself have an ethical dilemma? (A personal moral obligation to keep herself safe related to unsafe working conditions, versus her professional ethical obligation to meet the health and safety needs of patients in Ethiopia.)

❏ What is the role of unsafe working conditions in the dilemma?

❏ Is the nurse's family made better off by her emigration?

5 **Distributive justice**

❏ What are the Ethiopian government's responsibilities to its citizens regarding health and safety?

❏ Is it ethical for developed countries to recruit nurses actively from less-developed (in terms of money as well as number of nurses to care for the population) countries?

❏ Does it depend on the resources within Ethiopia?

❏ What role does the export of nurses play in the economic well-being of the people of Ethiopia?

❏ Does the decrease in nurses to provide care endanger the health and safety of Ethiopian citizens?

❏ Taking patient safety into consideration, is international recruiting of nurses an ethical practice?

CONCLUSION

Countries need to meet the healthcare needs of their population. International recruitment of nurses seems inevitable in this age of globalisation. There are positive aspects as well as challenges and opportunities related to the migration of nurses. It is incumbent on every country to implement a workforce plan that includes effective recruitment and retention of nurses, as well as meeting its economic needs with the resources at its disposal. With scarce resources, this is not an easy task. It seems that whenever there is a shortage of something valuable, it is more appreciated. I hope that a positive outcome of the global nursing shortage is more empowerment of nurses, leading to better working conditions, improved patient safety and better financial rewards.

REFERENCES

Aiken L, Clarke S, Sloane D, *et al*. Hospital Nurse Staffing and Patient Mortality, Nurse Burnout, and Job Dissatisfaction. *Journal of the American Medical Association*. 2002; **288**: 1987–93.

American Public Health Association. *Ethical Restrictions on International Recruitment of Health Professionals to the US*. 2005. Available at: http://www.apha.org/programs/globalhealth/section/advocacy/globalihtest2.htm (accessed 22 June 2007).

Beauchamp T, Childress J. *Principles of Biomedical Ethics*. 5th ed. New York: Oxford University Press; 2001.

Buchan, J. Global Nursing Shortages Are Often a Symptom of Wider Health Systems or Societal Ailments. *British Medical Journal.* 2002; **324**(7340): 751–2.

Buchan J, Calman L. *Global Shortage of Registered Nurses: an overview of issues and actions.* Geneva: ICN; 2005.

Buchan J, Sochalski J. The Migration of Nurses: trends and policies. *Bulletin of the World Health Organization.* 2004; **82**(8): 588.

Buerhaus P, Staiger D, Auerbach D. Implications of an Aging Registered Nurse Workforce. *Journal of the American Medical Association.* 2000; **283**(22): 2948–54.

Carney B. The Ethics of Recruiting Foreign Nurses. *The Catholic Health Association US.* 2005; **86**(6): 31–5.

DH, UK. *Guidance on International Recruitment.* 1999. Available at: http://www.dh.gov. uk/prod_consum_dh/groups/dh_digitalassets/@dh/@en/documents/digitalasset/ dh_4034794.pdf (accessed 22 June 2007).

DH, UK. *Code of Practice for NHS Employers Involved in the International Recruitment of Health Professionals.* 2004. Available at: http://www.dh.gov.uk/en/Publicationsandstatistics/ Publications/PublicationsPolicyAndGuidance/DH_4097730 (accessed 22 June 2007).

Herdman E. Globalization, Internationalization and Nursing. *Nursing and Health Sciences.* 2004; **6**: 237–8.

HRSA. *Human Resources and Services Administration Nursing Workforce Study.* 2005. Available at: http://bhpr.hrsa.gov/healthworkforce/reports/publichealth/default.htm (accessed 22 June 2007).

ICN. *Ethical Nurse Recruitment Position Statement.* 2001. Available at: http://www.icn.ch/ psrecruit01.htm (accessed 22 June 2007).

ICN. *Patient Safety Position Statement.* 2002. Available at: http://www.patienttalk.info/ pspatientsafe.htm (accessed 22 June 2007).

Kohn L, Corrigan J, Donaldson M, editors. *To Err is Human: building a safer health system.* Washington: National Academy Press; 1999.

Meleis A. Brain Drain or Empowerment? *Journal of Nursing Scholarship.* 2003; **35**: 105.

National Patient Safety Foundation. *Agenda for Research and Development in Patient Safety.* Chicago, IL: National Patient Safety Foundation; 2000.

Needleman J, Buerhaus P, Mattke S, *et al.* Nurse-staffing Levels and Quality of Care in Hospitals. *New England Journal of Medicine.* 2002; **346**: 1415–22.

Needleman J, Buerhaus P. Nurse Staffing and Patient Safety: current knowledge and implications for action. *International Society for Quality in Health Care.* 2003; **15**(4) 2275–7.

Seloilwe E. Globalization and Nursing. *Journal of Advanced Nursing.* 2005; **50**(6): 571.

Singh J, Nkala B, Amuah E, *et al.* The Ethics of Nurse Poaching From the Developing World. *Nursing Ethics.* 2003; **10**(6): 666–70.

US Bureau of Health Professions. *Projected Supply, Demand and Shortages of Registered Nurses, 2000–20.* 2000. Available at: http://www.ahca.org/research/rnsupply_demand.pdf (accessed 22 June 2007)

WHO. *The World Health Report 2006: working together for health.* 2006. Available at: http:// www.who.int/whr/2006/en/index.html (accessed 22 June 2007).

Xu Y, Zhang J. One Size Doesn't Fit All: ethics of international nurse recruitment from the conceptual framework of stakeholder interests. *Nursing Ethics.* 2005; **12**(6): 571–81.

19

How culture influences the reporting of unethical behaviour in the workplace

Faye Thompson

INTRODUCTION

Childbearing women have always sought culturally sensitive and competent care. In recent years, service providers and education programmes have also promoted this approach. Practitioners' narratives describe that working with women in a different cultural context opened their eyes and altered their 'way of seeing' (Thompson 2001, 2004). It also resulted in a conflict of values for them. Immigrant midwives bring with them the philosophy and values of their own culture, and decisions are made using interpretations based on these. What one group or individual deems as a reportable unethical incident, another may not. To what extent, therefore, does culture influence the reporting of unethical behaviour in the global midwifery-obstetric workplace? Disciplinary codes introduced in recent years to monitor the quality of nursing care in Western countries have been an important corrective instrument for serious professional misconduct (Hout *et al.* 2005). Although medication errors and unethical behaviour are closely linked, this chapters considers only the latter.

THE IMPACT OF POLICY ON MATERNITY SERVICES AND LISTENING TO WOMEN'S VOICES USING AUSTRALIA AS AN EXAMPLE

Obstetric practice in Australia requires that all pregnant women (indigenous and non-indigenous) living in rural and remote areas be transferred to a major town or city at 36 weeks' gestation and remain there until the baby is born. The rationale for this practice is to ensure what is seen as safety for mother and baby in the presence of (Western) medical care. There is, however, a lack of infrastructure to support women and families during this time, and it is only recently that research has begun to reveal the impact of relocation on the woman and her family.

Relationships and everyday lifestyle are disrupted. Frequently the woman has no support network around her during those last weeks. Indigenous women are often housed in hostels, where they feel unsafe because of the presence of alcohol and violence, and when they do come into labour they have to get themselves to a hospital sometimes several kilometres away; and usually by taxi, which is an added financial cost.

The relationship between mothers and older children (indigenous and non-indigenous) deteriorates because the children feel that the mother left them, and when she returns with a new baby it takes a considerable period of time to rectify the disrupted relationship, as well as develop a good relationship between the older siblings and the new baby. For many women living in rural and remote Australia, this means that the family income/business suffers because both partners are needed to work the farm or property. Children's schooling is disrupted because rural women spend several hours a day teaching their children literacy, mathematics, and the humanities, including cultural values.

In earlier research (Thompson 2001), I recorded the following scenario. Gemma, a non-indigenous midwife practising on an island off the Australian mainland, said:

> When they [the indigenous Australian women] came back to the island, of course they would often just 'go to ground' till they were almost ready to have their babies and they'd turn up on the clinic doorstep in the middle of the night and produce their babies – usually quite well without any problems and that was a real difficulty because I personally had a problem with sending these women back all the time over to the mainland when I knew that that's not where they wanted to be and there were really no suitable mechanisms in place to support them over on the mainland . . . basically if they came in and had their babies we just supported them – we didn't say much to them at all.
>
> Yes it did open my mind to thoughts that there is another way. I had to think hard about what I'd been taught – about safety, about the issues involved, the very hospital training that I had and where it fitted into all of that and it is a conflict when you first start challenging those beliefs . . .
>
> It had a really positive effect on me personally because up until then I'd been fairly much a hospital-oriented midwife believing that the only place to have a baby was the safety of a hospital and all that sort of nonsense, and those women taught me that that's not so.

Two other key issues arise. The first is practical and political: it is not only the individual practitioner's ethical behaviour that needs our attention but institutions, infrastructures and systems also warrant close scrutiny for their ethical adequacy and impact on individuals. The second issue, although philosophically based, also has very real and practical implications: 'What must something be like in order to qualify as a subject of serious moral concern in its own right?' (Winkler 1993, p. 353).

Kay was a white mother who also participated in the earlier research (Thompson 2001). She considered that her wishes were not heard or respected and she was not able to establish realistic expectations for her birthing experience:

> As we [private practice female obstetrician and mother] met throughout my pregnancy I would raise the subject of wishing to have as natural a childbirth as I could manage and the conversation didn't develop on that. It was quickly switched to other issues, not related necessarily even to the birth [for example, which private school the unborn baby would attend]. Very little time was spent discussing the birth.

Kay eventually had an unplanned caesarean section birth for this first baby. Disappointed and dissatisfied with her first experience, she sought midwifery supervision for her second pregnancy and birth, and progressed with no narcotic medication or obstetric intervention to a vaginal birth of a healthy baby in a hospital setting with only her private midwife in attendance. To avoid their disapproval, Kay lied to her immediate family about the supervision of the second pregnancy and she told them that she was visiting a doctor.

Does Kay's former type of relationship, with its lack of engagement, qualify as a subject of serious moral concern in its own right? How were the obstetrician and pregnant woman each defining and interpreting the concepts of autonomy, self-determination and informed choice? The way we see or interpret our social world greatly influences how we are and act in that world. Tension and conflict may arise, for instance, in clinical decision making, and reporting of mistakes and behaviour, when practitioners view childbirth and their role in that process from differing philosophies of care (Way 1998).

To what extent did the dominant healthcare culture influence the reporting and non-reporting of those two circumstances? Who would Gemma, the midwife, and Kay, the pregnant woman, go to with their complaints? To whom should they report or disclose what they 'saw' and considered to be 'not ethical' behaviour? Kay commented that she saw the hospital midwives as powerless: certainly not as advocates for her. Rather than being encouraged to provide feedback and express concerns, individuals such as childbearing women, and in some circumstances midwives, are at best kept ignorant of processes and persons for reporting and, at worst, are actively discouraged from speaking out against the dominant culture. This is accentuated for vulnerable immigrant people who find themselves without a common language or shared understanding of the cultural and contextual values and beliefs.

Gemma met several times with her nurse-midwife superiors in the government Health Department. She explained that all nursing staff on the island were also registered midwives, and sought a change of policy to allow indigenous women on the island to 'birth on their country' in keeping with their cultural beliefs, values and practices; but little changed, and after some years Gemma moved away from the area.

Rosemarie Tong (2000) asks if we have the necessary conceptual tools to achieve a global ethics that creates unity in and through our diversity. Feminist ethics is a possibility because it aims to eliminate or modify systems, structures, and sets of norms that contribute to human oppression, particularly women's oppression. Striving for sameness, however, can result in human oppression: moral absolutism and colonialism. Conversely, an overemphasis on respect for difference can fail to confront some social injustices. Global bioethics is therefore only possible if we continually look for wrongdoers and oppressors with all our senses, emotion and reason, not simply with blind justice, and if we are partners in virtue and friends in action, sharing meaningful goals and tasks in common.

MEANING AND DIMENSION OF 'MORAL COMPETENCY'

One commonly used definition of culture is 'the learned, shared and transmitted values, beliefs, norms and life-ways of a particular group that guides their thinking, decisions and actions in patterned ways' (Leininger 1991, p. 147). Moral competency in nursing is said to be the individual's ability to live in a manner consistent with a personal moral code and role responsibilities, necessary because decision making and advocacy in nursing and midwifery practice depend on technical knowledge, values, beliefs and ethics (Jormsri *et al.* 2005).

Mothers and midwives have shared values in relation to ethics surrounding childbirth (Thompson 2001, 2004). The use and abuse of power, a relationship, context, and virtues such as moral character are recurring features in their narratives. Institutional dominance characterised by paternalism, lack of self-determination, a fear and mortality-morbidity focus, and being unsupportive of women with a procedure-oriented approach was rejected by both groups as ethically inadequate or incompetent in the present discussion.

Intentions inform behaviour, and are situated in narrative histories within particular settings. These mothers' and midwives' narratives identify the practitioner's intention, and tell us how intentions differ in particular settings, even within the same culture.

There is a broad moral consensus that we should do something about wrong behaviour or else have good and specific reasons for not doing anything. Integral to this is our culture and interpretation of the context.

MEANING AND USE OF THE CONCEPTS 'ADVOCACY' AND 'DISCLOSURE' IN THE CONTEXT OF WESTERN MATERNITY SERVICES

Advocacy arises out of the ethic of caring and rests on humanity, needs and rights between people in any given relationship.

Systems are often criticised for causing the condition that requires advocacy in the first place and then ridiculing the advocate for questioning authority. Focusing on individuals as advocates starts a process of blame, and there is no effective infrastructure for fixing what is really wrong, i.e. the cause of the error or misbehaviour.

Tom O'Connor and Billy Kelly (2005) indicate that nurse advocates act primarily as intermediaries between patients and healthcare environments, that this places the nurse advocates in conflict and confrontation with others, and that this can be detrimental to the nurse advocates both professionally and personally.

The institutional culture impacts on disclosure to patients (Tuckett 1998). Whistleblowing is defined variously as the act of revealing something covert or informing against another, or identifying an incompetent, unethical, or illegal situation in the workplace and reporting it to someone who may have the power to stop the wrong (Peternelj-Taylor 2003).

Moral metaphors are culturally determined, highlighting certain features of experience while suppressing others. Advocacy metaphors conceal potential moral conflicts because they suggest that advocates act on behalf of only one party instead of cooperatively between people of equal position, thus implying that other healthcare practitioners somehow do not act in the patient's best interests (Thompson 2004).

Non-disclosure of information to patients is widespread and justifiable because nurses attempt to avoid the harmful effects of distress on their clients (Teasdale & Kent 1995). According to Anthony Tuckett (1998), registered nurses (a) make a clear distinction between lying and deception; (b) choose to lie, deceive or tell the truth when the client is benefited or prevented from harm and depending on the situation; and (c) emphasise the relationship with another when choosing to lie, deceive or tell the truth. The nurses' role and the institutional culture of the workplace influence decisions about lying and deception. Professionals are more likely to report a colleague's behaviour or practice when written protocols provide them with strong grounds, and less likely to report 'behaviour that has negative consequences for the patient when that behaviour reflects either compliance with a protocol or improvisation where no protocol is in place' (Lawton & Parker 2002, p. 17). An English survey of obstetricians and midwives found that:

> Views on the necessity of reporting the 10 designated obstetric incidents varied considerably. For example, 96% of staff stated they would always report a maternal death, whereas less than 40% would report a baby's unexpected admission to the Special Care Baby Unit. Midwives said they were more likely to report incidents than doctors, and junior staff were more likely to report than senior staff. The main reasons for not reporting were fears that junior staff would be blamed, high workload and the belief (even though the incident was designated as reportable) that the circumstances or outcome of a particular case did not warrant a report (Vincent et al. 1999, p. 13).

Earl Winkler's (1993) question remains relevant: what must something be like in order to qualify as a subject of serious moral concern in its own right?

DISMANTLING THE 'BLAME' CULTURE

We need to understand why people fail to report concerns and develop systems and cultures that make disclosure (discussion and reporting) easier. The concept of accountability is frequently related to that of responsibility as '[a]ccountability through information disclosure is a cultural practice closely associated with the emotional state of guilt' (Velayutham & Perera 2004, p. 52).

Incident-reporting behaviour also differs between medical and nursing professional groups. For example: 'Nurses reported more habitually than doctors due to a culture which provided directives, protocols and the notion of security, whereas the medical culture was less transparent, favoured dealing with incidents "in-house" and was less reliant on directives'; and in relation to the culture of blame, focus-group participants suggested an 'option to report anonymously to an independent body, without fear of being identified and with the option to omit identifiers of either self and/or organization, and education' (Kingston et al. 2004, pp. 36, 38).

A Queensland study (Walker & Lowe 1998) found that attention to individuals rather than to processes results in nurses having a genuine fear of reprimand from those in authority if they report an incident and, therefore, are reluctant to identify themselves on incident forms. Correctly, complaints of negligence and sanctions by disciplinary boards are patient-centred.

Liz Hart and Jenny Hazelgrove (2001, p. 257) question the usefulness of the term 'conspiracies of silence'. They suggest that 'cultural censorship' better describes 'how adverse events get pushed underground, only to flourish in the underside of organisational life'. Understanding attitudes towards reporting concerns is essential if the conspiracy of silence or cultural censorship is to be altered because, according to Jenny Firth-Cozens *et al.* (2003), attitudes are having a real effect on whether or not people do report their concerns. Nurses who report misconduct at work suffer severe physical, emotional and professional consequences and, while those who remain silent in the face of misconduct do not experience professional problems, like whistle-blowers, they experience many physical and emotional problems (McDonald 1999).

Using a meta-analysis of previously published results, Wen-Chin Li *et al.* 2007) demonstrated statistically significant differences between Taiwan, India, and the US in human factors contributing to aviation accidents. Differences were related to organisational processes, organisational climate, resource management, inadequate supervision, physical and mental limitations, adverse mental states and decision errors; factors mostly concerned with higher organisational levels and style of management rather than operation of the aircraft per se. Could a meta-analysis of healthcare 'accidents' produce similar results?

Critical incidents from 200 registered nurses in the US revealed tensions they faced when attempting to adhere to policy while managing the realities of their everyday professional lives (Orbe 2000). According to Naresh Khatri and Jonathon Halbesleben (2007), management control and focus on immediate hazards produces a culture of blame; an employee-participation approach produces a culture of learning from mistakes, camaraderie and motivation.

USING A CULTURALLY SHARED UNDERSTANDING TO PROMOTE DISCLOSURE AS POSITIVE

Valuing diversity and embracing global similarities will help to create understanding about why people fail to report concerns and to learn from mistakes.

Attempting to decrease culturally inherent differences amounts to 'acculturation', and 'acculturation implies learning new behaviors in addition to language that may conflict with previous cultural practices' (Miller & Chandler 2002, p. 27). A culturally shared understanding would not result in acculturation, or focus on profiles of particular groups. All of these have the 'tendency to overemphasize culture and normalize beliefs for specific ethnic groups [for example, all Spanish speaking] . . . Important differences within groups are ignored at the expense of presenting a homogeneous cultural unit with a set pattern of beliefs and values' (McGrath 1998, p. 18). The approach deflects attention away from influencing social factors and institutional forces. Rather, as Barbara McGrath (1998) and Shigeko Izumi (2006) propose, understanding will bridge the gaps. Cultural competency means understanding the culture, so that one can think through the purpose of, and beliefs embedded in, the observed behaviour. This enables us to interact with one another in an educated and appropriate way. It is critical to explore and identify one's own values and beliefs, and to understand the real-life ethics that is overlooked by universal Western philosophical ethics (Izumi 2006; Thompson 2004).

Approaches to, and the status of, nursing, midwifery and other healthcare services around the world are not all the same. What is common to nurses and midwives is the value of providing quality care. By being mindful of the values that individuals across cultures hold in common, we can overcome some of the challenges of integrating diverse perspectives into that care. Across cultures we have a universal desire to live up to our best values, and to do this we need to *really* listen to each other 'by learning about other ethical perspectives, engaging in ethical listening and opening the heart' (Cameron 2006, p. 312).

DIVERSITY AND SIMILARITY

Diversity is a reality. Diversity can be seen in all cultures.

'Whilst women giving birth in the developed (sic) world focus on fetal well-being and the quality of their birth experience, those women living in the developing (sic) world face the harsh reality of high maternal and infant mortality rates . . . Working within the framework of traditional birthing practices and utilizing lay midwives who are well respected in their villages is proving effective in reducing infant mortality caused by tetanus' (Callister 2001, p. 210). Probably 80% of the world's babies are born at home. Yet, any women who enter the US healthcare system are expected to enter the hospital and give birth according to US standards, while being cared for by nurses, midwives and others who may not understand their cultural values and beliefs surrounding pregnancy and childbirth (Ottani 2002).

Given that this is the experience of consumers of maternity care, what are the implications for immigrant nurses and midwives who are also expected to enter the workforce in their host country, adopt local values, and practise according to local codes and regulations?

WORLDWIDE PHENOMENA

There are at least six worldwide phenomena that consistently appear and that allow practitioners to cross cultures in daily encounters with clients by focusing on similarities (Giger & Davidhizar 1995):

1   communication
2   social organisation

3 space/touch
4 time
5 environmental control
6 biological variation.

Can these phenomena be utilised within our organisations, infrastructures and policies to promote disclosure of unethical behaviour as positive?

Communication: Value observation and listen to more than the spoken word. Be aware of, and understand the significance of how people communicate, tones of voice, and so on.

Social organisation, space and touch: 'Observe the proximity of family members to one another and to the labouring woman' (Ottani 2002, p. 35) and note if this is congruent with the behaviour of the practitioner(s). Review the language used. Feminists and constructivists agree that language and discourse not only reflect social organisation but they also construct our identity and subjectivity (Wurzbach 1999). Policy makers can benefit from learning about culturally insensitive and unethical 'mistakes' and 'misunderstandings', through narrative feedback. More flexible and inclusive guidelines can be developed that not only assure high-standard healthcare but also support differing world views, and assist in minimising conflict experienced by either immigrant or 'native-born' staff.

Time: Recognising the Western preoccupation with clock and calendar time may mean that we in the Western world develop a shared understanding of the importance, or not, of the passage of time. The Western interpretation of a 'missed' event may constitute an 'error' for one party while it is quite unimportant to another party concerned with meaningful and culturally competent relationships.

Environmental control: Creating a comfortable birthing environment for herself, the birthing woman is a global phenomenon. The claim that 'Nurses and other care providers need to observe, listen, and ask . . . [and] value another's values' (Ottani 2002, p. 35) may be so idealistic, however, as to be impractical. A code of ethics or professional conduct that requires the practitioner to 'value another's values' or 'respect the cultural values and practices of the other' may become a punitive instrument if it is deemed that the (immigrant or native-born) practitioner has not demonstrated similar values to the 'other' or has not facilitated practice of them. Local law and/or policy may even make the latter action illegal or deserving of disciplinary action. Attention to individuals rather than to processes results in nurses having a genuine fear of reprimand from those in authority if they report an incident (Walker & Lowe 1998). There is usually little demand on institutions or infrastructures to be accountable for providing support of differing world views or a work environment that supports the midwife's decision making. Western culture relates accountability to responsibility, which in turn is associated with the state of guilt, and the latter is most frequently directed towards the individual.

As one participant in the study by Charles Vincent et al. (1999) suggested: 'Could we encourage reporting of difficult situations that were well-handled?' (p. 19). Tanja Mander and Sven Staender (2005) claim, in their discussion on open disclosure, that effective communication between healthcare providers, patients and their families is an important element of how adverse events and their aftermaths are handled.

CONCLUSION

Although the need for open disclosure is acknowledged throughout the literature, and much has been written on whistleblowing in clinical practice, there is little discussion on the extent to which culture and the globalisation of nursing and midwifery influence reporting of unethical behaviour in the workplace.

Globalisation has implications not only for consumers but also for immigrant nurses and midwives, who are expected to enter the workforce in their host country, adopt local values and practise according to local codes and regulations. Developing a shared global understanding that embraces diversity and similarity will minimise risk to both consumers and practitioners (immigrants and native-born).

Global bioethics is possible only if we continually look for wrongdoers and oppressors with all our senses, and if we share meaningful goals and tasks. By understanding the values that individuals across cultures hold in common, we can overcome some of the challenges of integrating diverse perspectives into our commonality, i.e. the care we provide. Our universal desire to live up to our best values requires us *really* to listen to one another and dismantle the blame culture.

Finally, the question is posed once more: what must something be like in order to qualify as a subject of serious moral concern in its own right?

REFERENCES

Callister LC. Culturally Competent Care of Women and Newborns: knowledge, attitude, and skills. *Journal of Obstetric, Gynecologic and Neonatal Nursing.* 2001; **30**(2): 209–16.

Cameron M. Nursing Ethics: listening to each other. Report of ICNE and *Nursing Ethics* conference, Taipei, Taiwan, 19 May 2005. *Nursing Ethics.* 2006; **13**: 304–12.

Firth-Cozens J, Firth RA, Booth S. Attitudes to and Experiences of Reporting Poor Care. *Clinical Governance.* 2003; **8**: 331–6.

Giger J, Davidhizar, R. *Transcultural Nursing: assessment and intervention.* 2nd ed. St. Louis, MO: Mosby Year Book; 1995.

Hart E, Hazelgrove J. Viewpoint: understanding the organisational context for adverse events in the health services: the role of cultural censorship. *Quality in Health Care.* 2001; **10**: 257–62.

Hout FAG, Cuperus-Bosma JM, Huben JH, van der Wal G. The Disciplinary Code for Nurses and its Contribution to the Quality of Nursing Care in the Netherlands. *International Journal of Nursing Studies.* 2005; **42**: 793–805.

Izumi, S. Bridging Western Ethics and Japanese Local Ethics by Listening to Nurses' Concerns. *Nursing Ethics.* 2006; **13**: 275–83.

Jormsri P, Kunaviktikulm W, Ketefian S, Chaowalim A. Moral Competence in Nursing Practice. *Nursing Ethics.* 2005; **12**: 582–94.

Khatri N, Halbesleben JRB. Relationship Between Management Philosophy and Clinical Outcomes. *Health Care Management Review.* 2007; **32**: 128–39.

Kingston MJ, Evans SM, Smith BJ, Berry JG. Attitudes of Doctors and Nurses Towards Incident Reporting: a qualitative analysis. *Medical Journal of Australia.* 2004; **181**(1): 36–9.

Lawton R, Parker D. Barriers to Incident Reporting in a Healthcare System. *Quality and Safety in Health Care.* 2002; **11**: 15–18.

Leininger M. *Culture, Care, Diversity and Universality: a theory of nursing.* New York: National League for Nursing; 1991.

Li WC, Harris D, Chen A. Eastern Minds in Western Cockpits: meta-analysis of human factors in mishaps from three nations. *Aviation Space and Environmental Medicine.* 2007; **78**(4): 420–5.

Mander T, Staender S. Aftermath of an Adverse Event: supporting health care professionals to meet patient expectations through open disclosure. *Acta Anaesthesiologica Scandinavica.* 2005; **49**: 728–34.

McDonald S. Whistleblowing: effective and ineffective coping. *Nursing Forum.* 1999; **34**: 4–13.

McGrath BB. Illness as a Problem of Meaning: moving culture from the classroom to the clinic. *Advances in Nursing Science.* 1998; **21**(2): 17–29.

Miller AM, Chandler PJ. Acculturation, Resilience, and Depression in Midlife Women From the Former Soviet Union. *Nursing Research.* 2002; **51**: 26–32.

O'Connor T, Kelly B. Bridging the Gap: a study of general nurses' perceptions of patient advocacy in Ireland. *Nursing Ethics.* 2005; **12**: 453–67.

Orbe MP. Negotiating the Tension Between Policy and Reality: exploring nurses' communication about organizational wrongdoing. *Health Communication.* 2000; **12**(1): 41–61.

Ottani PA. Embracing Global Similarities: a framework for cross-cultural obstetric care. *Journal of Obstetric, Gynecologic and Neonatal Nursing.* 2002; **31**(1): 33–8.

Peternelj-Taylor C. Whistleblowing and Boundary Violations: exposing a colleague in the forensic milieu. *Nursing Ethics.* 2003; **10**: 526–38.

Teasdale K, Kent G. The Use of Deception in Nursing. *Journal of Medical Ethics.* 1995; **21**: 77–81.

Thompson FE. The Ethical Nature of the Mother–midwife Relationship: a feminist perspective. [Unpublished PhD dissertation]. Toowoomba, Queensland, Australia: University of Southern Queensland; 2001.

Thompson FE. *Mothers and Midwives: the ethical journey.* Oxford: Elsevier; 2004.

Tong R. Is a Global Bioethics Possible as Well as Desirable? A millennial feminist response. In: Tong R, Anderson G, Santos A, editors. *Globalizing Feminist Bioethics: crosscultural perspectives.* Boulder, CO: Westview Press; 2000. pp. 27–36.

Tuckett A. 'Bending the Truth': professionals' narratives about lying and deception in nursing practice. *International Journal of Nursing Studies.* 1998; **35**: 292–302.

Velayutham S, Perera MHB. The Influence of Emotions and Culture on Accountability and Governance. *Corporate Governance.* 2004; **4**(1): 52–64.

Vincent C, Stanhope N, Crowley-Murphy M. Reasons for not Reporting Adverse Incidents: an empirical study. *Journal of Evaluation in Clinical Practice.* 1999; **5**(1): 13–21.

Walker SB, Lowe MJ. Nurses' Views on Reporting Medication Incidents. *International Journal of Nursing Practice.* 1998; **4**(2): 97–102.

Way S. Social Construction of Episiotomy. *Journal of Clinical Nursing.* 1998; **7**(2) 113–17.

Winkler ER. From Kantianism to Contextualism: the rise and fall of the paradigm theory in applied ethics. In: Winkler ER, Coombs JR, editors. *Applied Ethics: a reader.* Oxford: Wiley; 1993. pp. 343–65.

Wurzbach ME. The Moral Metaphors of Nursing. *Journal of Advanced Nursing.* 1999; **30**: 94–9.

SECTION 7

Summary

20

Globalisation and the future: some conclusions

Verena Tschudin and Anne J Davis

THINK GLOBALLY, ACT LOCALLY

The catchphrase 'Think globally, act locally' has been used in many situations, but reputedly was coined by the NGO Friends of the Earth in 1969.

There is inevitably a significant tension between the local, which is known and easily accessible, and the global, which can be remote and even alien. Knowing how best to use and benefit from both systems is crucial for good care to be accessible for patients and nurses, as care will increasingly be given at home and on the spot. It is even more crucial to know the local and global values, concerns, offers, possibilities and rights in healthcare in particular, but in community living in general.

In our world, every living system starts small and expands. This is as true of biology as of industry and commerce, and of weather systems as of relationships. Perhaps the exception is the idea of globalisation. The starting point here is that a global market exists, and gradually everyone will benefit from it. This top-down structure works well if all players have the same values and similar world views, play by the same rules and have the same conditions to begin with. As is now clear, and the chapters in this book have shown well enough, this is far from the case, and many of the hoped-for and proclaimed advantages of globalisation also have significant disadvantages, leading to loss and suffering.

Human beings thrive in an environment where they can be in charge of their world, which is usually their own surroundings and involves a fairly limited number of people. It is also in such situations that personal and professional values are formed, fostered and disseminated. Values affect the structures of small and large organisations, but are often implied, becoming clear only when they are challenged. With globalisation, many local and previously unacknowledged values have surfaced all over the world.

David Landes (1998) argues that whether or not a country copes well with globalisation depends how 'outward' (i.e. globally oriented) or 'inward' (i.e. inward-looking) its culture is. In inward-looking countries it tends to be the women who come off least well, because such countries find it difficult to 'foster adaptability and adoptability' (Friedman 2005, p. 412). This implies that such countries may have adopted a stance of 'me against the bad world', whereas outward-looking countries adopt a stance of 'the more of us together all over the world, the better'. The inward stance reduces the playing field to a few (often shadowy and mainly male) people who tend to defend their own values, subjecting their own people's values to their own. When traditional local values are questioned and are no longer seen as relevant, the whole structure of the known world begins to be doubted. Values need to grow from trust among some people, to be validated by a wider circle, and only then can they be accepted by larger groups. In the globalised world, everything depends on huge networks of people and interests functioning together to be successful. Nowhere is this more obvious or necessary than in healthcare.

HEALTHCARE SYSTEMS

We are now so used to rapid changes and advances in healthcare that we may forget that both of them rest on research, experiments, trials, and often a great deal of misery until something better surfaces. Globalisation has enabled innovations and practices to be shared with people around the globe within minutes.

Governments decide on the kind of healthcare systems a country has and how this is paid for. All such systems are increasingly seen as financial, economic and global businesses and enterprises. While they exist for the health of the nations, they may also be profitable to shareholders, depending on their funding sources and operational ideologies. Large international businesses tend to attract criticism because the larger the business, the less transparent they become, and it can be difficult to establish if all parts of an international business are accountable to the local situation. It is arguable whether healthcare systems should ever be managed for profit. National governments generally protect their control over healthcare, but a large part of that depends on other international conglomerates, such as pharmaceutical companies and technological and scientific hardware suppliers.

Healthcare is also part of a nation's concern, together with stability, security, education and general infrastructure, as these elements tend to be at the mercy of large global events, such as wars, conflict, terrorism, natural disasters (e.g. earthquakes and climate extremes), migration and labour force movements. It therefore becomes clear that any healthcare system is more than a national enterprise. The spread by vectors of formerly fairly localised diseases, such as malaria, dengue fever, West Nile virus, and so on, is a clear sign that globalisation also has different – and not always beneficial – effects.

The topic of labour migration has been well addressed in this book, and needs to be seen in the wider context not only of direct healthcare, but also of the stability of populations. People who migrate leave behind a vacuum where other family members may need to step in to care for dependants, where grandparents may need to act as parents, or men to care for children. This may involve role changes that are uncomfortable, and may lead to psychological morbidity. Traditional health and social care systems may not be able to cope with such situations, leaving nations destabilised, leading to internal unrest. Globalisation as an ideology was unable to foresee these possible downsides in its drive for 'bigger and better'. All nurses, however, have firsthand experience of caring for people who became victims of systems they knew nothing about and had no power to change. Nurses alone cannot change such systems, but nurses have the possibility and responsibility to address such effects where they become aware of them, initially by listening to stories told by people for whom they care. Through research into causes and effects of situations they meet, they are at the cutting edge of reducing suffering of many kinds.

A large amount of attention has been paid to the demographic reasons for labour migration, i.e. the increased demands made on healthcare systems by better conditions and interventions in the West and North, and the ageing population worldwide, including the ageing labour force. These issues need to be acknowledged as part of the whole concept of the globalisation of nursing, and they are regularly addressed in the international press.

Healthcare systems serve not only patients and ill people, but also have a wider role in preventive care. Indeed, the first responsibility for nurses mentioned in the ICN *Code of Ethics for Nurses* (2005) is 'to promote health'. The remit for this is wide and may range from personal instruction for a patient, to national campaigning for certain health-promotion issues. As an example, at the time of writing, all primary school children in Scotland are receiving free school meals for a period of six months in 2007–08 (British Broadcasting Corporation 2007) with the aim of making children aware of the need for healthy eating to combat illness in later life. Scotland, although a well-developed country, has very high rates of diet-related diseases. In this instance, the health needs of an entire nation are considered, not simply certain diseases or groups of people, demanding coordination with many agencies, such as healthcare, education, food supply, finance, advertising, as well as the staff needed to put such projects into action.

The growing use of surgery via video-linkup, of robots and telecare, have potentially huge implications for care in remote places, for responding to accidents or disasters where the right skills are not available at the right time, and for pioneering work. The armed forces in many countries are significant users of such equipment in field hospitals, where the expertise eventually translates into care at home. Given the present ease of communication, medical and nursing discoveries and advances can be disseminated so that many people can benefit easily. A small idea or innovation can quickly gain acceptance; conversely, large companies often need to work together (and not be concerned about competition) to trial some innovation in very small settings and work with local people to achieve best results. Globalisation in healthcare, and in particular in technology, increasingly challenges accepted practices and logic by crossing boundaries of time and space, and traditional ways of thinking and acting. The issue may be whether such applications are the right or best use of resources at the right time; i.e. the ethical questions about the use of resources also need to be asked and answered by nurses, who use increasingly sophisticated technology.

A GLOBALISED FUTURE NURSING

Findings from the WHO (2002) indicate that much of future healthcare will be long-term, home-based care. Demographic calculations predicting longer life for increasing numbers of people worldwide, and better healthcare generally, have lead to these conclusions. While people live longer, they also stay healthy much longer and elderly people are not significantly more prone to ill health than younger people, given that life-style illnesses (obesity, diabetes, heart disease) tend to affect younger people as much as the older population. These diseases do not require hospital care; rather they demand that the people affected by them are better educated in dealing with their conditions themselves instead of being in constant need of expert nursing care. Thus a different type of nurse may be called for in situations of long-term, home-based care.

Nurses may need to act more as heath consultants than as practising carers, with more family members and trained assistants involved in the daily care. Increasingly in the more affluent countries, people prefer to have their babies at home, die at home (Marie Curie Cancer Care 2007), and are more quickly discharged back home after hospital interventions. Medical advances have enabled much treatment to be given on the spot in walk-in centres, by nurses, and as day surgery. With the increase of hospital-acquired infections, people prefer not to go to hospitals and, as hospital-based care becomes more specialised and shorter, the global healthcare system will need to be changed drastically in the near future.

The impact on nursing of such changes is inevitably huge. For some time, the argument has been made that 'generalist' nurses will be needed in future (Tschudin 1999). Given that most care will concentrate in the home in future, many more nurses will be needed in community care. Such nurses may need to be educated differently, have different views of healthcare, and be able to function in a significant number of roles. We still use the term 'healthcare' when mostly we mean the care of sick people. It seems ironic that we so often distort the meaning of certain things by the way we speak about them. The word 'nurse' is another example. The word is related to the Latin *nutrire*, which means to nourish, giving a strong link to 'educate' in the sense of bringing up children. In the future scenario of nursing, seeing nurses as educators and carers, who accompany people over a time to enable them to become experts in their own disease and disease management, seems very relevant. In this sense, it would then also be more relevant to speak of 'healthcare' and indeed mean what the word conveys.

Such an understanding of healthcare may imply that nurses working in the community in future may have a decisive role in community building. The globalisation of markets has to be balanced with the localisation of values and needs. Acting locally does not foster exclusivism; on the contrary, as local communities (especially in the West and North, where communities are not strong at present) will increasingly be made up of people from many cultures and with many values and beliefs, new communities have to be formed and values discovered and fostered. Nurses working in community settings have to be adept at inter-agency work. If they are to 'educate' healthy and sick people in life-long health and care, nurses need to be familiar with issues of schooling and education, jobs, transport, police, industry, business, leisure and many other local concerns for their clients to flourish in the locality. It is only in local settings that local policies can be initiated. Indeed, while they may be networking and dealing all day with global colleagues, people may increasingly need and want to spend their leisure time in their own home and pursue locally generated activities. The global does need to be balanced with the local for psychological and spiritual well-being.

Nurses seem to be the professionals with the most immediate relevance to be concerned about local issues simply by the broad clientele they serve. Thus nurses may also be the professionals who can best understand the necessary local values, which may then be understood very broadly as: promoting health and well-being; preventing physical, mental and emotional illness; restoring health and community; and alleviating suffering of many variations. These aspects would give the four responsibilities of nurses described by the ICN (2005) a much more holistic meaning.

An example of a system where this is to some extent functioning already is Slovenia. This small country has a system of community nurses caring for families, rather than individuals. One nurse visiting a house may have to care in different capacities for a newborn baby and the mother, a teenager after a minor accident, give advice to a middle-aged person on some aspect of care, and assess an elderly person's dementia. This system is unique but very effective, and appreciated by the population. It may well be an example of how healthcare systems in the future may need (and want) to make use of nursing personnel. It may also be something that the nursing profession may want to consider as a possible way of giving nursing as a profession a realistic sense of professional importance, and the local community an appropriate system of care that combines the ICN's fundamental responsibilities of nurses of promoting health, preventing illness, restoring health and alleviating suffering (ICN 2005).

Communities are fluid entities and in order to flourish, a great deal of give and take is necessary. Local communities reflect what is happening in the global community; when local communities are cohesive and productive, a huge network of relationships is created, which may act in the global interest. There is no doubt that a great wave of re-ordering, re-thinking and re-creating is under way in most areas of our lives at present, much of it caused by globalisation and advances in technology. The meaning and value of culture and community, and their expressions, depend largely on what individual people and local communities are willing to make and share with others, for the good of the whole. Nursing as a profession may be a very important player in this. Since care of some kind will always be needed. With the changing care needs it will depend on how such caregivers are valued and rewarded. Nurses who are dispersed more and therefore less visible in the community, rather than visible and concentrated in hospitals, may suffer from being devalued by governments concerned with short-term financial returns. Hence it is imperative for the nursing profession to have a strong voice in local, national and international policy formation.

Nursing education will, of necessity, have to adapt. Most often it is practice that shapes theory, rather than the other way round. Theory has a very important place in helping us understand concepts but, if theory cannot be applied in practice, there is no place for it. If nurses have to learn multi-tasking much more than at present, including working effectively in inter-agency situations, then nurse education will also need to change soon. Given that it takes three to four years of basic education, and another five or six years of practice to attain expertise, education for a different future has to start now. Teachers of nurses need to learn the new skills and ways of thinking and functioning first; something that is not achieved overnight.

Certain knowledge, such as the basics of anatomy and physiology, seems to be necessary for all nurses to function intelligently. Beyond that, it largely depends on the type of work any nurse is engaged in as to what else is necessary for practice. Nursing organisations have been considering the future of nurse education and various models are available (ICN 2007). For these reasons, it is necessary to understand the local situation, needs and values.

Education always seems to lag behind developments, but projections can, at least to some extent, contribute to the changing requirements. The growing need for skilled and partially skilled nursing personnel to work in the care of older people is inevitably growing, and therefore needs to be addressed. This, in turn, needs a fundamental assessment of attitudes to older people, at least in Western and Northern countries. In these countries, older people are often shunned and not valued, therefore people do not want to work with them either. In Eastern and Southern countries of the world, where cultural mores favour communities rather than individualism, older people tend to be given the status of 'elders', endowed with wisdom and leadership. With nurse migration, and nurses being deliberately trained 'for export' in various Asian countries, the cultural differences and adaptations may need a great deal of understanding and experience, if discrimination is to be avoided.

Most of all, nurse education needs to prepare for work in the community and it needs to be much more flexible than at present. A great deal of nurse education is possible via electronic means, including virtual classrooms, and television and video linking. An element of education that can never be replaced is group discussions, where much of the emotional learning takes place, but good study material can also be created to learn the more intangible subjects, such as interpersonal, communication and social skills. With many of these means of teaching, good imagination in how to use the material and the equipment is essential. Indeed, imagination (a form of empathy) is one of the most important personal assets for anyone wanting to teach.

Flexibility of mind and practice may increasingly be needed when adapting to global living, as globalisation will constantly demand new ways of knowing, living and working. The rapid changes in almost all areas of life that have become the norm means that people who are not flexible, who cannot imagine a different future, or who have limited education, will find it increasingly hard to fit into a global system that demands the opposites of these.

The role of nursing organisations is crucial in much of this work, as it is mainly those associations that have the necessary professional and political voice for large numbers of nurses. On the whole, national nursing associations are also respected by governments, precisely because governments can then talk with elected representatives of the profession. Many national organisations and associations also combine with other health professional bodies on certain policy issues that concern them all, to strengthen the nurses' voice.

BEING INVOLVED GLOBALLY

In a globalised world there is never going to be only one good way of dealing with any subject, and whatever can be said here may be relevant for one reader, and not for another, simply because situations and circumstances vary. The ethical basis for a globalised nursing workforce is also a point in question. Most of us concerned with ethics and nursing have long learned that one particular theory or one specific set of principles is inadequate. Instead, it is useful to look at any subject from various points of view. This has the disadvantage of not being able to be called 'authoritative' and therefore perhaps being relative, but it has the advantage of being undogmatic and more fitting to any given situation. What this second approach needs is the capacity to listen and be empathic. An approach based on these two human ways of being and behaving is likely also to be compassionate, which most people will appreciate as genuine. Indeed, this fits well with a care ethics or a feminist ethics, both of which have often been described as being more appropriate to nursing and healthcare generally than any other ethical framework.

Responsibility

One aspect of ethics is always responsibility. It is perhaps significant that we often speak of the responsibility that healthcare professionals have, but rarely of their rights; and that we often speak of the rights patients and clients have, but rarely of their responsibilities. With a slight distortion of the way the word is written in English, responsibility can point us to the *ability* to respond. Without diminishing here the concept of incompetence, anyone who is competent also has the ability to respond. This includes responding appropriately to any given situation, which may be a delighted, critical or sorrowful response, depending on the circumstances. It may also be an unreflected or instinctive response, and maybe one that is regretted later. To be human and express humanity, however, there is a need to respond constantly in life to any action upon us. The first need is *that* we respond; the second is *how*.

In a possible future where nurses may be taking on many more roles and work across many boundaries, and perhaps more in the original sense of the word 'nurse', it would seem important that nurses foster in their clients a 'self-management . . . to provide a substantial opportunity to find self-determination in primary and ongoing care that the normal focus on the clinic does not afford' (Kukla 2005, p. 37). Patients and clients will need a great deal of information to care better for themselves, and they will need to be acting responsibly towards themselves and this information. Nurses and patients will share much more equally the rights and responsibilities of care and, indeed, of living well and healthily. For this reason, responsibility will enhance self-determination, but seen within relationships in family and local community. A globalised future is not able to function if people consider only 'me, my and mine'; indeed, the wider concept of globalisation has quickly shown that we are much more dependent on one another than we may perhaps like or even desire. With healthcare being huge global systems, and healthcare personnel often from many different cultural and ethnic groupings to the ones they serve, we need to think much more in terms of 'us, our and ours'. Responsibility is the symbol of such arguing and acting, as it stems from listening and leads to compassion.

Most countries have aid projects in areas of the world where there is a need for help, support, education and innovation. The list would be too long, but Canada, Japan, and Taiwan should be mentioned (websites) as generous donors. However, it is the people on the ground who make the difference, not money alone. Many nurses who have been on exchange programmes return with different attitudes and recognise global responsibilities in which they want to be active (*see also* Chapter 16). By being involved, they see wider and further, and are personally challenged in how to live as human beings and also in how to foster responsibility in others. The concept of social justice becomes something to consider more seriously; to understand its basis, what is needed to reach its goals, and how these goals have also a personal element of responsibility.

The value of nursing

Within nursing, some of this may be expressed in how the profession is willing to be challenged by new circumstances, and how creatively it is willing to reply. Globalisation has forced us to 'think globally'. Rather than be frightened by this, the profession as a whole – and indeed many other professions, as well as industries and businesses – need to look into the future and try to see what can be put there. Nurses need a wide vision in which they are able to hold together the small and the large, the local and the global. Their concern needs to be for a society where peace and stability are possible.

All significant moves are made by people who have a clear vision, and are not afraid to go against the prevailing wind or cross boundaries and remove obstacles that seem immovable. This takes courage, but courageous acts encourage others. A good deal of this is being done already, especially by the ICN (2007), but it is also necessary that individual nurses do not leave all the work to the international nursing association, as even the ICN can function only on what happens when people 'act locally'. It is the local action that informs the global thinking.

The value that nursing has in the eyes of governments and policy makers depends largely on the value that nurses themselves give it. When looking at nursing as a profession with the eyes of governments, they may consider mainly the costs of highly qualified people, of efficiency, and the effectiveness of staff. They are not concerned with individual relationships between nurses and patients, and with values such as 'care', 'respect', and 'dignity' that nurses themselves find difficult to define and that cannot translate directly into monetary values. It is therefore perhaps not surprising that nursing as a profession often gets short shrift and is considered as marginal. Good care can also be given by less experienced people, or with the help of technological devices that do not need a salary. Nurses therefore need to make it very clear that nursing is an indispensable profession. This is why not only a clear vision is needed, but also evidence of how this vision will function in the future; and *all this needs to be said and heard in the places where it matters*. For this reason, the idea of responsibility takes on a much wider meaning, and one that is not a burden, but a challenge and a reward.

Philosopher Alfred Whitehead considered that people have a threefold urge: 'i) to live, ii) to live well, and iii) to live better' (1929, p. 8). Within a framework of globalisation and responsibility, the demand for 'homo ethicus' is surely to consider all three seriously, and how to put them into practice.

What individual nurses can do

- Consider what local values you hold, and why.
- Discuss these with work colleagues and refine them, to understand their relevance and significance, and yourself (your team) in relation to them.
- Be aware of local and national issues in healthcare, education, social life, and so on.
- Join a nursing organisation that is able to speak for you and take an active part in it.
- Make concerns known locally and nationally.
- Write to the local press about local concerns.
- Lobby your member of government, NGOs, watchdog organisations.
- Keep records and/or a diary of important issues or events. Nothing impresses policy makers more than giving them evidence.
- Join Internet chat rooms and social forums
- You have a voice; use it. You have an important contribution to make; make it. You can change the world around you; act locally and globally.

REFERENCES

British Broadcasting Corporation. 2007. *Schools Begin Free Meals Scheme*. Available at: http://news.bbc.co.uk/1/hi/scotland/glasgow_and_west/7054334.stm (accessed 23 October 2007).

Friedman TL. *The World is Flat: the globalized world in the twenty-first century*. London: Penguin; 2005.

ICN. *Code of Ethics for Nurses*. Geneva: ICN; 2005.

ICN. *Islamabad Declaration on Nursing and Midwifery*. 2007. Available at: http://www.icn.ch/Islamabad_Declaration.pdf (accessed 1 November 2007).

Kukla R. Conscientious Autonomy: displacing decisions in health care. *Hastings Center Report.* 2005; **35**(2): 34–44.

Landes D. *The Wealth and Poverty of Nations.* London: Time Warner Books; 1998.

Marie Curie Cancer Care. *Delivering Choice Programme.* Briefing note, 19 November 2007. Available at: http://www.mariecurie.org.uk/NR/rdonlyres/D744E789-F459-4B9D-B841-51F0100FC5F1/0/briefingnotek241.pdf (accessed 27 November 2007).

Tschudin V. *Nurses Matter: reclaiming our professional identity.* Basingstoke: Macmillan; 1999. (particularly chapter 9, 'Nurses as moral artists', pp. 178–95).

Websites: http://www.acdi-cida.gc.ca/aideffectiveness; http://www.mofa.jp/policy/oda/guide/1998/5-2.html; http://www.news.vu/en/news/inter/041202-the-taiwan-side.shtml (accessed 27 November 2007).

Whitehead AN. *The Function of Reason.* Boston, MA: Beacon Press; 1929.

WHO. Current and Future Long-term Care Needs. WHO/NMH/CCL/02.2. 2002. Cited in Hirschfeld M. An International Perspective. In: Davis AJ, Tschudin V, de Raeve L, editors. *Essentials of Teaching and Learning in Nursing Ethics: perspectives and methods.* Edinburgh: Churchill Livingstone; 2006. pp. 325–37.

Index